A farmer's life for Me

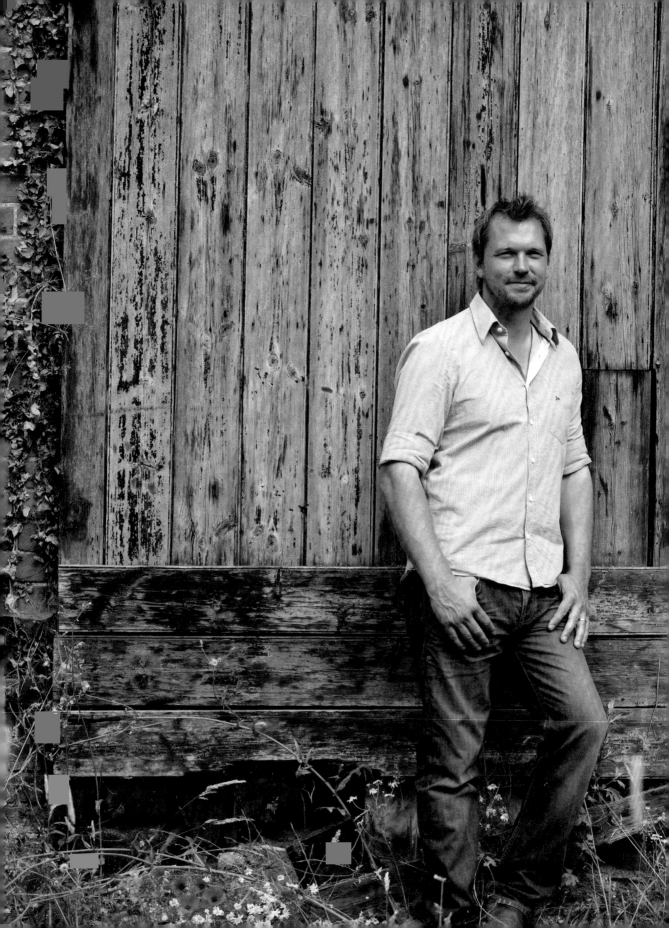

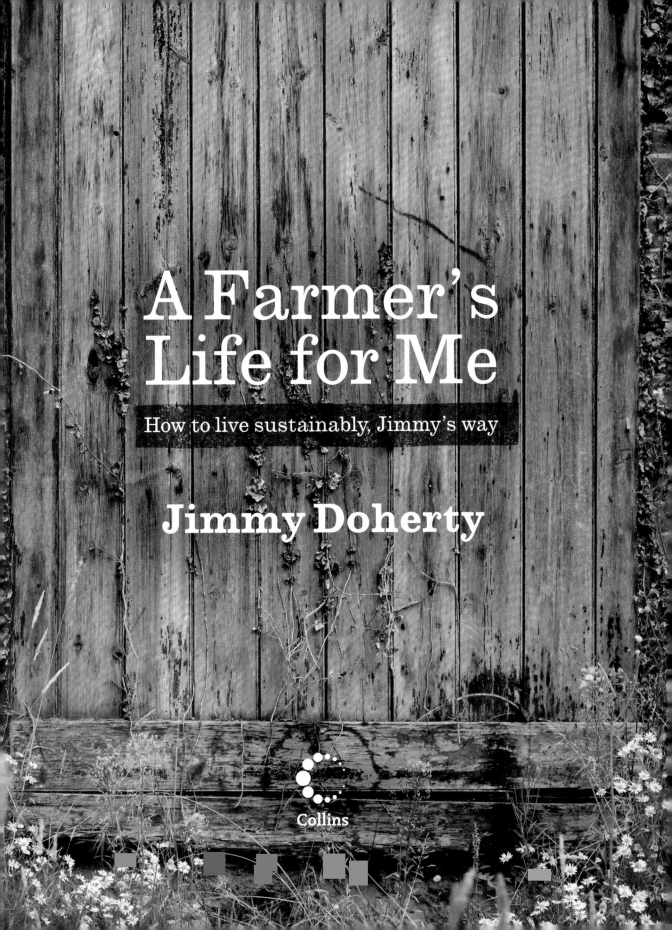

A Farmer's Life for Me

How to live sustainably, Jimmy's way

Jimmy Doherty

Collins

Dedicated to my beautiful wife Michaela and Molly Rose.

First published in 2011 by Collins, an imprint of HarperCollins Publishers

HarperCollins Publishers
77–85 Fulham Palace Road,
Hammersmith, London W6 8JB
www.harpercollins.co.uk

10 9 8 7 6 5 4 3 2 1

BBC and the BBC logo are trademarks of the British Broadcasting Corporation
and are used under licence. Logo © BBC 1996

Text © 2011 Jimmy Doherty
Photography © 2011 Chris Terry
Illustrations © 2011 Debbie Powell

Jimmy Doherty asserts the moral right to be identified as the author of this work

A catalogue record of this book is available from the British Library

ISBN 978-0-00-741195-5

Printed and bound by Butler Tanner and Dennis Ltd, Frome, Somerset
Design – Smith and Gilmour
Editorial director – Jenny Heller
Editor – Helena Caldon
Production – Stuart Mascheter
Illustrations – Debbie Powell, The Artworks
Food styling – Anna Jones

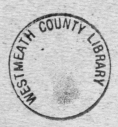
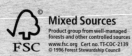

Mixed Sources
Product group from well-managed
forests and other controlled sources
www.fsc.org   Cert no. TT-COC-2139
© 1996 Forest Stewardship Council
FSC

FSC is a non-profit international organisation to promote the responsible management
of the world's forests. Products carrying the FSC label are independently certified to
assure consumers that they come from forests that are managed to meet the social,
economic and ecological needs of present and future generations.

Find out more about HarperCollins and the environment at www.harpercollins.co.uk/
green

CONTENTS

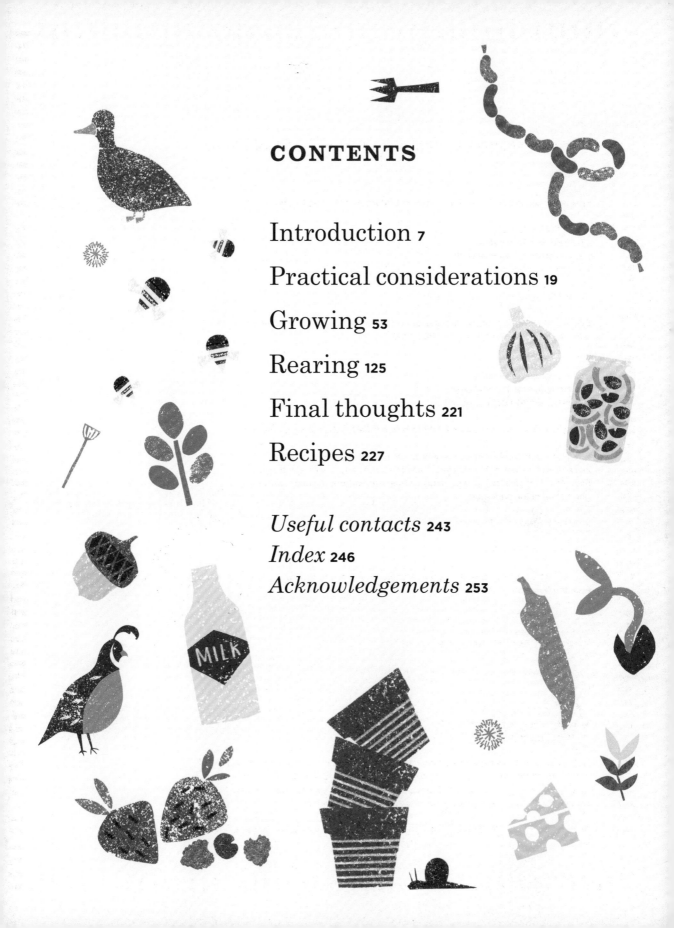

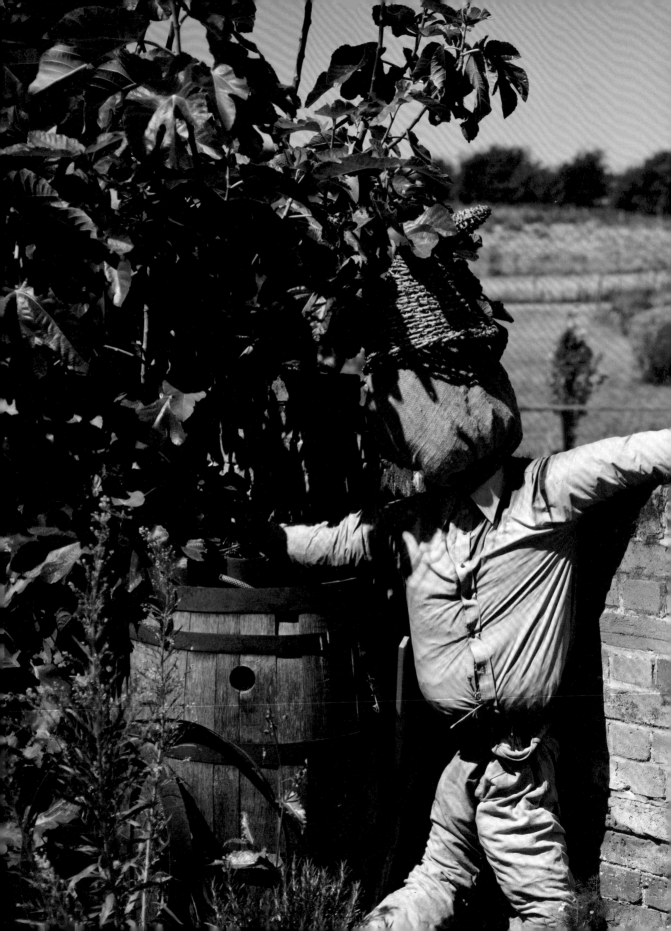

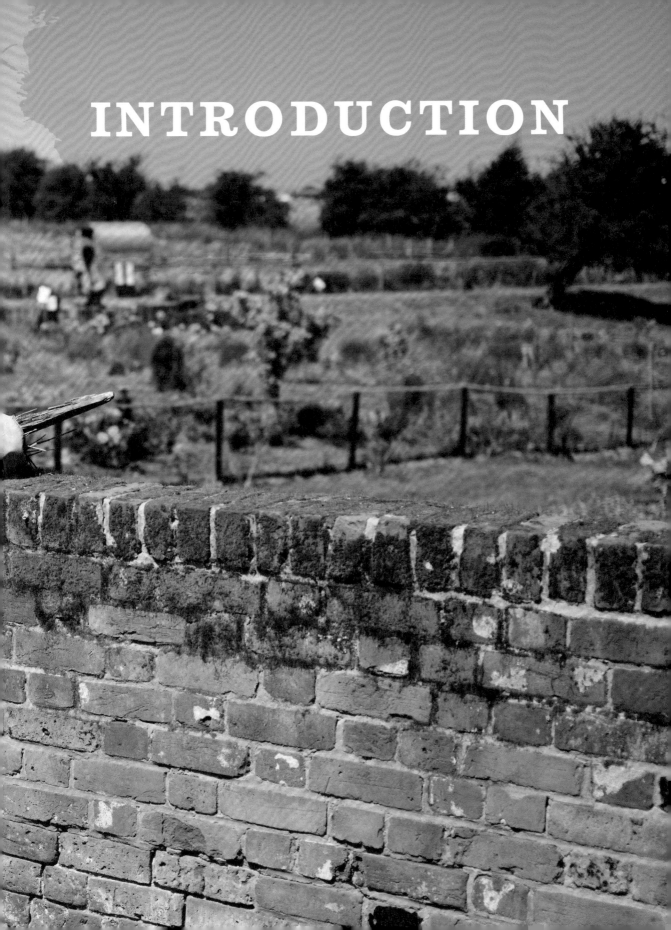

INTRODUCTION

'First came the SAUSAGE, then came the PIG'

I wasn't born in the country, but we moved to Saffron Walden when I was three. I grew up in what had once been a cricket pavilion, which my dad converted into a great little house surrounded by 2½ acres of meadow. As a toddler I pottered around the great outdoors. I loved animals from the very beginning and used to keep scores of them like some Essex version of Gerald Durrell. I had spiders and insects and ferrets and rabbits – I even converted the carport into an aviary.

The fields were even better, a never-ending source of interesting bugs and insects. My best friend had a smallholding – I saw my first lamb being born when I was 13 and the memory has stayed with me to this day – it was named Buttons! Later, I worked in a wildlife park in Widdinton, first as an assistant and then helping run the butterfly house. Attached to this was a working farm and it was that that kindled a real interest in farming.

But I buried that fascination for a while by heading off to do a zoology degree and then on to read for a doctorate in entomology. By the time I was in my mid-twenties I found myself teaching in Coventry and running the university insect lab. I was reasonably successful and broadly content, but something was missing.

What next?

It was 11 September 2001 that changed everything. I was staring down a microscope, counting flies, when the planes went into the Twin Towers. That event suddenly brought everything into perspective. I thought, what would happen if some calamity befell me? What if a car skidded off the road, if I was in a plane crash, or a scaffolding pipe fell onto me from a building as I was passing? What would my life mean? Would I just be a guy who one moment was counting flies and the next wasn't there any more? When people asked what I'd done with my life, would friends say, 'Jim? Oh, he counted flies'?

I had always had a deep-rooted respect for farmers. A lot of people just see a grumpy bloke in a flat cap complaining about the weather, but actually they are genuine wizards – the real Harry Potters and Dumbledores of today. They take an empty patch of ground and a few months later they've got the food we all rely on. You can't have a bank manager, computer programmer or politician without the farmer who produces the food we all need to survive. They've got rare skills, ones which we all rely on, and I can't bear the idea of losing this traditional knowledge.

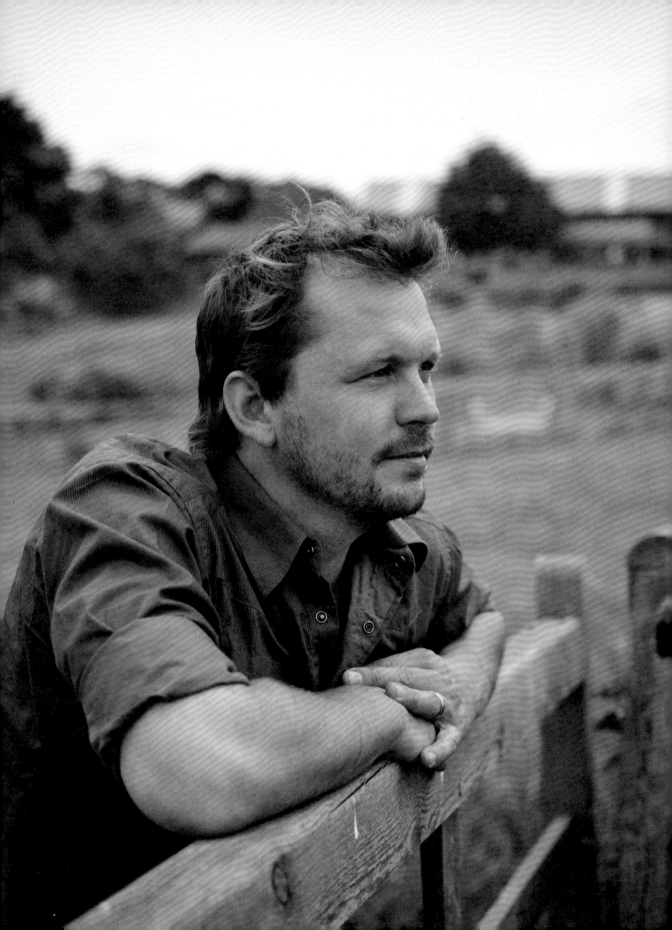

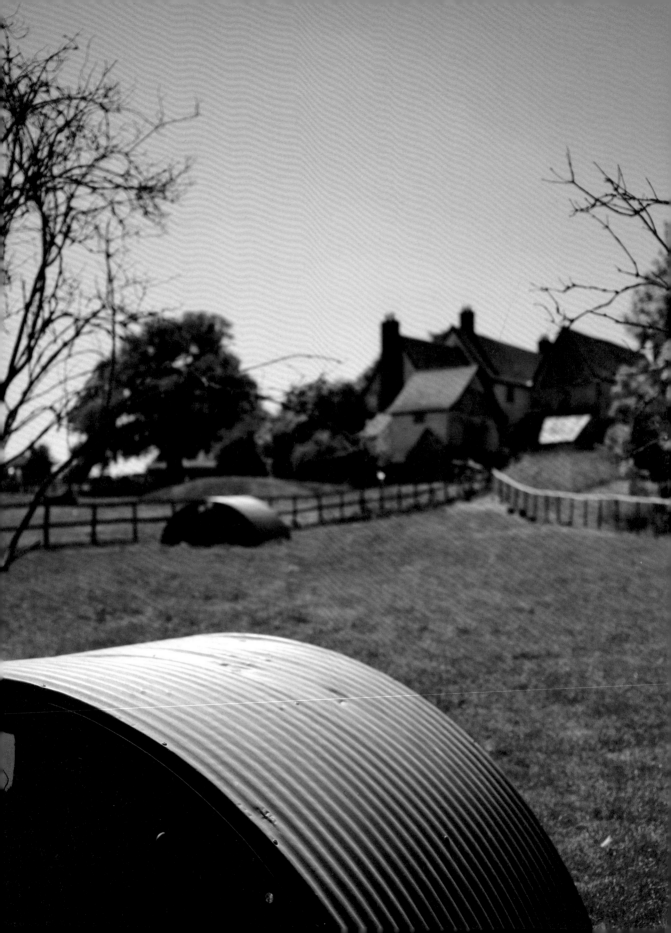

A future in farming?

So when I was looking around for something to do with my life, it seemed natural to turn to food production. My problem – and in some ways my great advantage – was that I had no farming background. This meant there was no father to turn to for help and no tractor to borrow, but it also meant I wasn't loaded down with years of doing things in a particular way and selling through the age-old channels of livestock markets and wholesale butchers. Instead I was free to experiment and make mistakes – and boy did I make some mistakes – and I could come at things from a fresh angle.

I knew there was no point in producing food without a market. I had no interest in growing and rearing things just as a self-indulgent hobby. In the end the only way you know you're doing a good job is if other people are prepared to pay for what you've produced. Our farm is very small in East Anglian terms, so it was clear I had to develop something unique, something that wasn't already out there. For my dreams to work, I knew I had to have a market.

I started by going to a lot of farmers' markets and then to Borough Market in London. All these are full of great producers with brilliant produce and really fantastic ideas. I looked at their stalls and I asked a lot of questions. To this day I am really grateful for the generous and incredibly helpful advice I got from countless producers who had much better things to do than answer my naive questions.

Pigs quickly struck me as ideal for what I wanted to do. They have large litters compared with sheep or cattle. In other words, each sow will produce at least eight piglets (we aim for ten in a litter), twice a year. A cow or sheep, on the other hand, will only manage one, or possibly two, young in the same period. Better still, you can keep them on very rough land, so it meant I didn't need a lot of expensive prime land. Pigs also mature quickly and are ready for slaughter at six months or so (it's at least two years with a beef animal). But, most important of all, they produce a fantastic meat which has a ready market in Britain. We just love our pork, bacon, ham and – of course – sausages.

Picking the perfect spot

I then started to look around for a farm. From the outset I knew that location would be critical. Someone once told me that it is really important to count the chimney pots that are visible from the farm – each one represents potential customers. I found the ideal location just south of Ipswich. It was an old farm in a poor state of repair with a few near-derelict barns, a stream or two and 100 acres of fairly rough pasture – the perfect place to rear pigs.

From the outset my pigs were always going to be reared outdoors. They like it and it's more natural for a start, but there are good practical reasons too. There's very little mucking out and they graze much more than people realise. This means they find a fair amount of their own food. They are also good at turning over rough ground. Admittedly, this does encourage thistles and docks, but you can get round that by ploughing and planting with crops or reseeding with grass.

Getting going

Once I had signed the lease on the farm, I started knocking things into shape. I began by putting up some rough-and-ready electric fencing. My first arks (movable runs) were no more than rudimentary straw bales with a waterproof top.

It was tough at first, but at least I always knew that to make a living I would have to add value in every conceivable way I could. Even the biggest pig farmers live on a financial roller coaster. Unlike cattle or sheep, there are no subsidies for pigs and the industry goes through regular booms and busts. If the biggest farmers were regularly going bankrupt, I knew I had to do something more than just produce pork – quality would be key. It was also vital to take control of as much of the journey from field to plate as possible. So while my first pigs were putting on weight in their paddock, I built a butchery out of old fridge panels inside one of the tractor sheds. It was crude, but the panels were virtually free and easy to wipe down and sterilise.

There is nothing wrong with modern commercial breeds of pigs – after all, they produce 99 per cent of the pork and bacon we eat in Britain today – but I wanted something extra special both in taste and texture.

It always strikes me as ironic that every major town has galleries and museums dedicated to preserving our artistic and cultural heritage, yet it's left up to a handful of unpaid enthusiasts to save our traditional breeds. These animals are the living embodiment of our agricultural past, and if they die out, that's it: they take their unique qualities and genes with them.

So I decided to buy up as many of the traditional East Anglian pig breed – the saddleback – as I could afford and establish my own herd. I consciously scoured the area looking for the last specimens from the old Essex lines and slowly I began to select some of the best gilts to build up our own breeding herd. Later I added other rare breeds – Tamworths, Berkshires and Gloucester Old Spots – each of which has its own particular virtues.

It was a good move. There's great character in their meat. It has denser muscle fibre and more fat for cooking, which makes it, in my mind, better meat, and therefore it's a more exciting eating experience too. Commercial pork has less resistance when chewed and the lack of fat means it has less flavour than its traditional cousins.

In the beginning it was just me and the butcher – and he doubled up as stockman

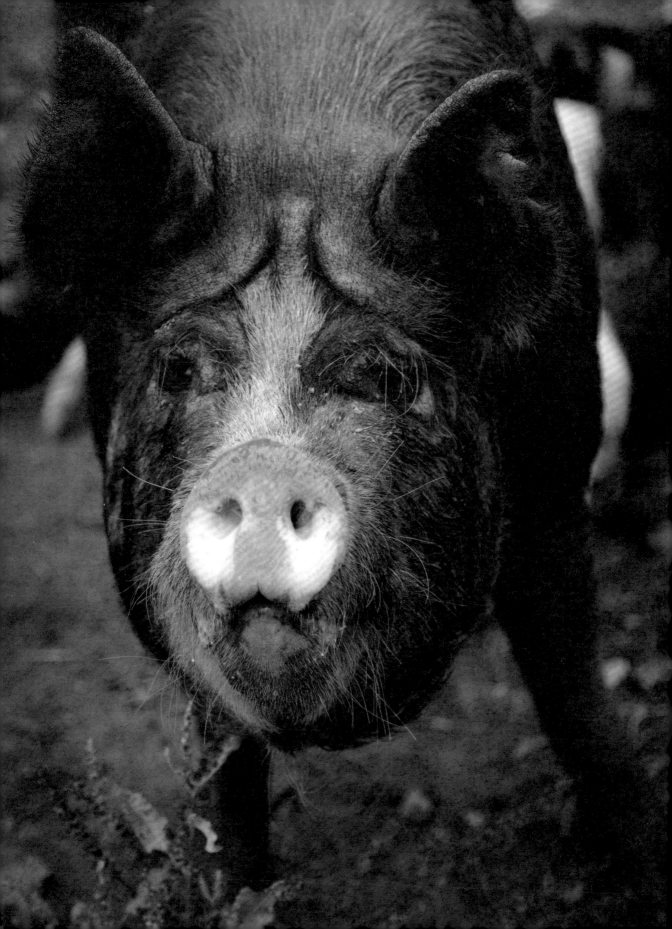

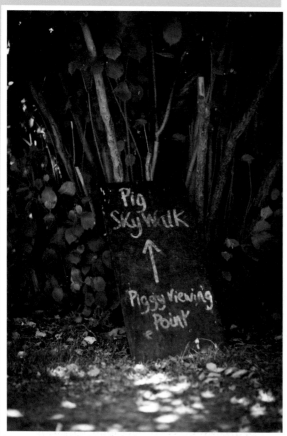

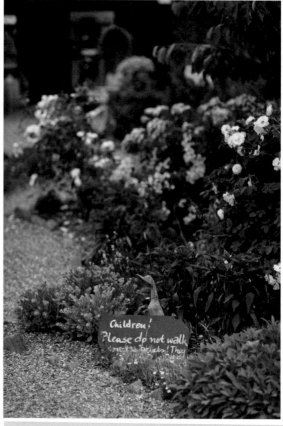

Children!
Please do not walk
on the borders! They...

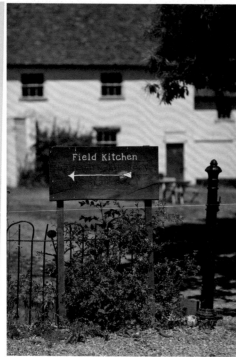

Field Kitchen

The BEST salesman
is the Person who
TRULY understands
the PRODUCT

when I was out at the markets. He was an ex-student of mine who, when he started, could just about remember how to cut things up, so he did all the butchery while I did the bacon – at least I did the bacon when I wasn't at one of the five various farmers' markets I was attending every week.

This was incredibly time-consuming, but looking back I know it was also vital. I just had to do the selling because I am convinced the best salesman is the person who truly understands the product. That generally means the farmer or the person who's turned it into something special and delicious. The other great benefit is that you get feedback. This is priceless for any producer; it's a chance to ask your customers what they like and what they don't like about your product. And then you take it on from there – what else do they like? What else would they like to see on your counter? It's a brilliant way to gather free and vital market research (no pun intended).

All the same, I slowly realised I couldn't do everything, so after a couple of years we started to employ a stockman. In fact, I think taking on too much is one of the biggest mistakes almost everyone makes when starting out with farming. They plant too much and then don't have enough time to water or weed it. Or they buy too much stock, forgetting that as it grows, so will its appetite and it will need ever-increasing amounts of expensive food, or more and more space.

Building the business

We decided to open the shop because we figured that there was always someone here anyway, so we might as well sell to anyone who turned up. When we had the official opening and we took £1,500 in a day I felt as if I'd won the Lottery. Naturally that dropped off a bit, but the important thing was that now people were coming to us rather than me spending a huge amount of time, money and fuel driving to farmers' markets all over East Anglia.

The next step was a natural one. When customers arrived to buy their sausages and pork, they were obviously keen to see the pigs. Once they'd seen the saddlebacks they wanted to compare them with the other rare breeds, so slowly we found the paddocks nearest the shop were turning into an animal trail. So I went out and bought a few rare breeds of sheep, cattle and poultry to make it more interesting, and then we got some rabbits and guinea pigs, a few ferrets, goats and a couple of rheas for the children.

We then turned one of the sties closest to the farm into a herb garden, and as people began to linger around it we put in a few bales for people to sit on and I got a cheap barbeque and cooked sausages. Most recently, I added something I had always dreamed of – a butterfly house. This is a polytunnel which is packed with exotic plants like bananas and ginger. It is full of the most beautiful tropical butterflies which fly around the visitors as they walk through. Next I want to

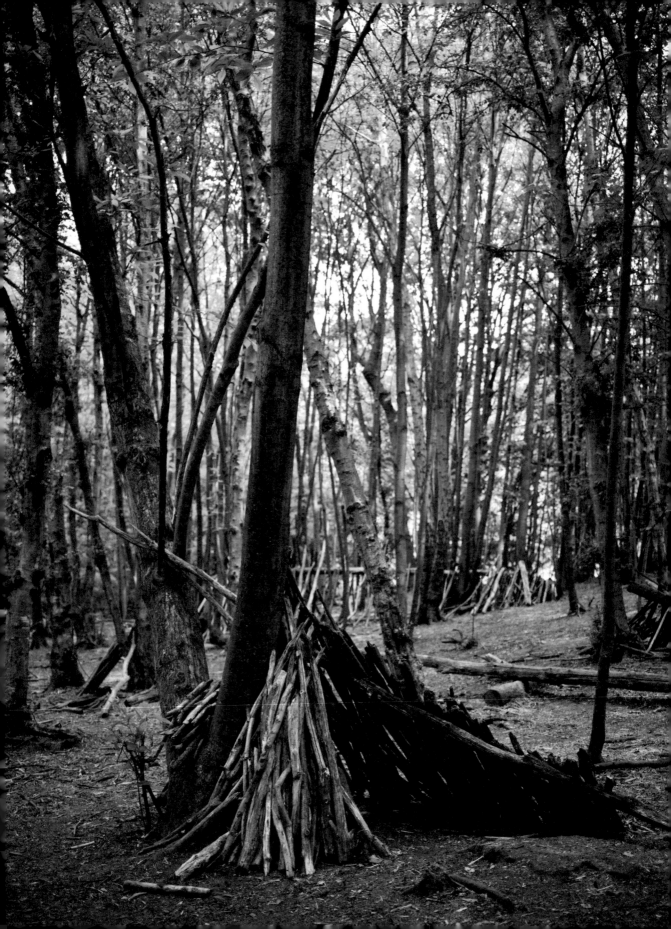

turn the adjoining paddock into a haven for British butterflies by encouraging wildflowers and food plants for the caterpillars.

All the way, as we slowly built up the business, we kept reinvesting every penny of profit. When I started I was so naive. In a way this was a good thing – it meant I went to see the bank manager full of confidence rather than weighed down with realistic predictions of what I'd actually be earning. My first business plans were all looking ahead at sales and they failed to take into account some of the elementary running costs. There is an accountancy saying: 'Profit is sanity, turnover is vanity' – but that's the trap most people fall into in their first couple of years of trading. They are thinking about the money coming into the cash tills and forgetting about the way money trickles out of the account day to day.

I carried on making mistakes, of course. For example, at the outset the online business was a mess. I muddled up the first two orders and sent each to the wrong address. Soon after we lost over £1,000 of produce when stock got delayed in transit, and while the courier will reimburse you for the carriage they don't cover perishable goods.

Looking back – and ahead

The whole journey from first arriving at the farm through the building up of the business has been great fun, with a lot of laughs. For example, just after we started the online business I was told the Prince of Wales had ordered 15kg of sausages. I was absolutely delighted. I thought he'd heard of the fantastic quality of my sausages and I had visions of 'By Royal Appointment' – can you imagine my disappointment when it turned out the Prince of Wales was the pub down the road?

I am still learning. No sooner do you get one new project running than fresh problems arise. No business is immune to the activities of the general economic climate, and this is certainly true of food production. A recession is a real test of a nation's food culture. One of the first things people cut back on is the quality of their ingredients. As a result takings at our weekly farmers' market have dived recently. At first this comes as a blow, but once I'd absorbed it I realised it could have advantages too. After all, it applies all the way up the food chain and actually the products that will really suffer are those at the top of the chain. My sausages are high-quality and not cheap as sausages go, but they are still very affordable. In other words, I reckon that if people are cutting back on fillet steak, then they are the perfect customers for a premium sausage instead. There's still a future in farming.

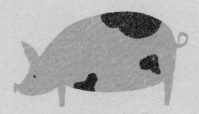

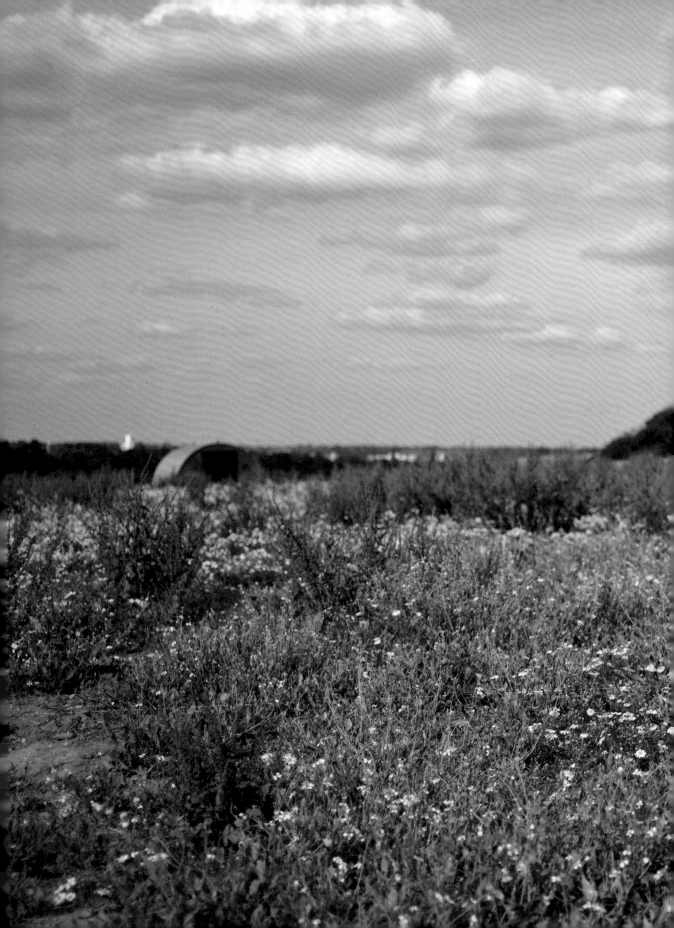

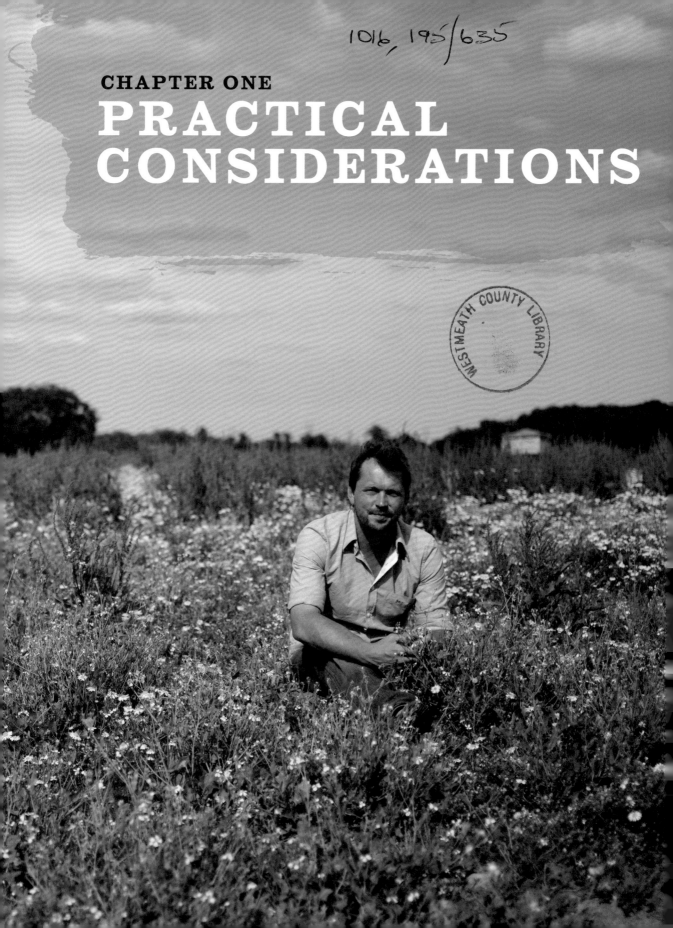

CHAPTER ONE
PRACTICAL CONSIDERATIONS

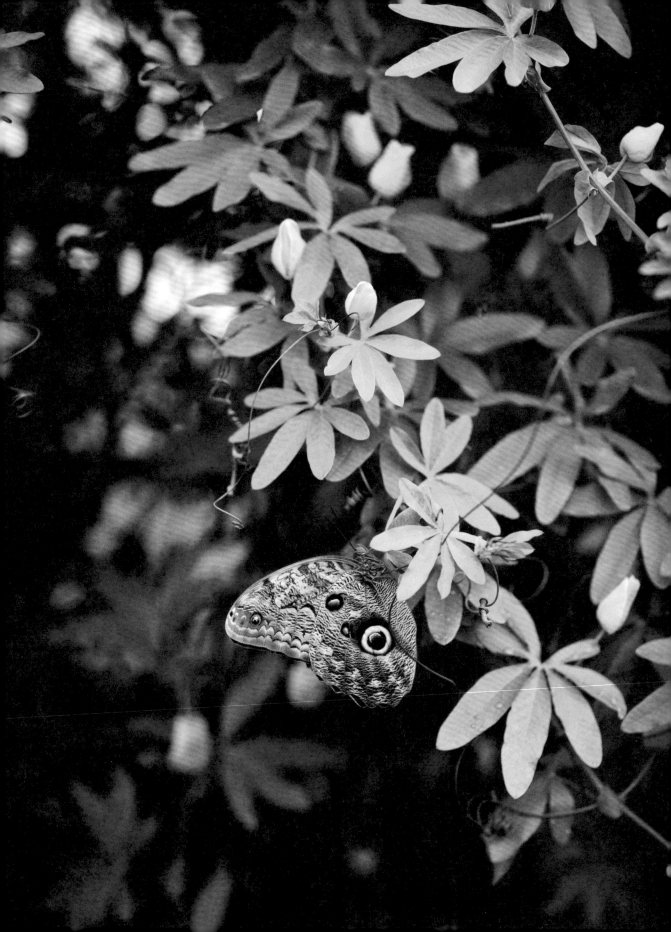

THE DREAM AND THE REALITY

BEFORE YOU BEGIN...

There is an intrinsic romance about farming. Perhaps it's something buried deep in our DNA, a long-lost urge to follow in the footsteps of our hunter-gatherer ancestors, but it seems as if almost everyone hankers after producing their own food.

This dream is very much alive today, and every year hundreds of thousands of people take their first tentative steps towards setting up their very own version of *The Good Life* by growing their first vegetables, collecting their first back-garden egg or tentatively bottling their first jam.

A few go further, 'seizing the day' to desert conventional nine-to-five urban life and set up in some rural idyll. Whatever route most appeals to you, the most important thing is to start by making some broad decisions; in particular, is this going to be a hobby or a career? If the latter, perhaps you should start in your spare time and then launch into it once you have learned the inevitable hard lessons and built up some experience.

Then there's the issue of what you are going to target: food or non-food, growing plants or rearing livestock? To make this work you need to enjoy this new venture, as you will probably need to put lots of time and effort into it, so it's fine to let your heart rule at the very outset. If you love working with animals but hate watering and weeding, then market gardening is probably not for you, but poultry or pigs could be the answer. If you love animals and are likely to build up bonds with them, then perhaps non-lethal farming –

such as eggs or specialist wools – might be less emotional than rearing for meat.

As a part of considering what it is that you are trying to achieve, you need to decide whether you want to produce just a little homegrown food to supplement your shopping or if you have grander dreams of being self-sufficient. Simply growing a few courgettes or gathering half a dozen eggs from your back-garden hens can be immensely satisfying; there is nothing like the warm glow of putting a home-produced meal in front of friends or family.

If you have bigger ideas and hope to sell your produce, you should decide whether you need to earn a living or if a little pocket money is enough. In either case, it's important to keep an open mind as you look at the possibilities. Remember – your ideas have to fit the market, not the other way round.

Let us assume that you do have a broad idea of what you want to do; the next step is to plan where you intend to do it. The budget you have available is clearly critical to the scale of your venture, but it is also often more flexible than you might think. Many small-scale schemes are perfectly feasible in cities, while other, grander ideas might require you to look further afield. Varying property prices across Britain mean that many homeowners do have the option of selling up their smaller space in the city and for similar money buying something much larger in the country.

For now, let's start at the beginning and see how best to turn the dream into a reality. If the whole idea of farming is new to you, it might be best to start small and gain that all-important experience before you commit to what will inevitably be a major life change.

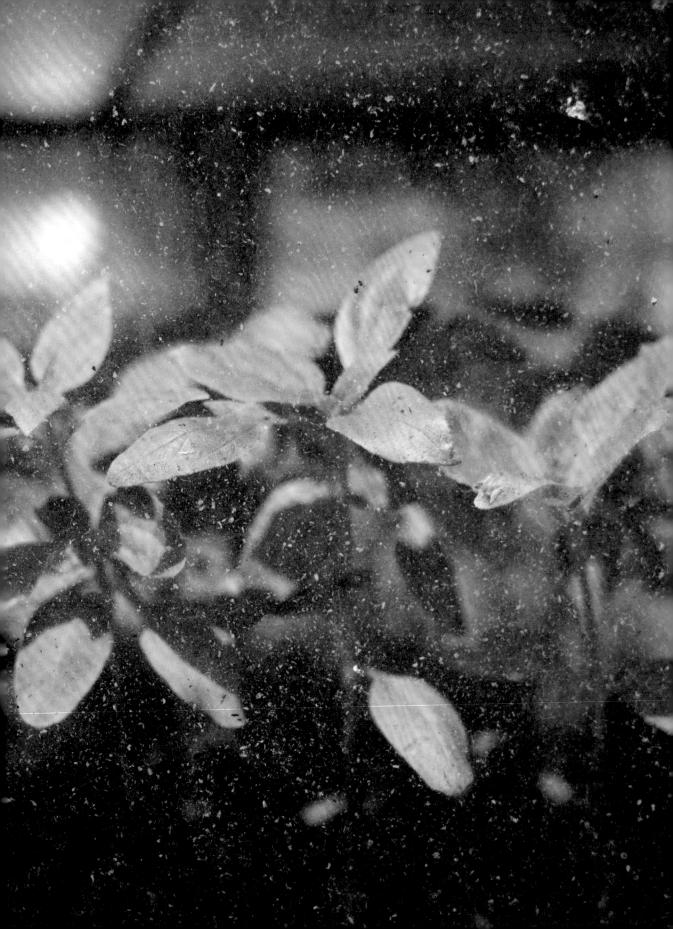

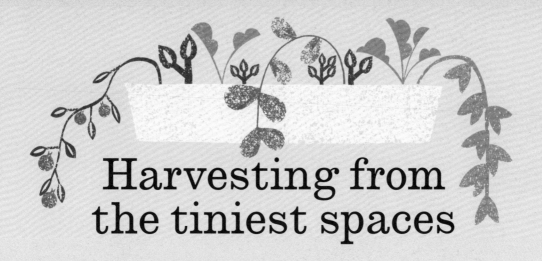

Harvesting from the tiniest spaces

Just because you dream of a kitchen stuffed with home-grown produce doesn't mean you have to sell up your city pad and move out into the countryside; it is perfectly possible to produce some food in the very smallest of spaces.

You can produce crops on windowsills, balconies or in hanging baskets, or you can even grow mushrooms and sprouting beans in cellars, under the stairs or beneath the kitchen sink, for example. Just two or three window boxes will provide all the fresh herbs most families will eat. If you have a balcony or a flat roof you could cultivate a more substantial amount of vegetables and fruit in growbags or tubs.

Another possibility that is often overlooked is house plants; instead of a yucca, for example, while not try growing a chilli plant? These are usually treated as annuals by most gardening books, but in their native tropics they are perennial shrubs – and most are very attractive too, particularly when festooned with colourful fruits.

There is a huge amount of fun to be had in the kitchen with your harvest,

and some of your produce could be turned to profit (it can often break even on the smallest scale). Markets, roadside stalls and pick-your-own farms are full of

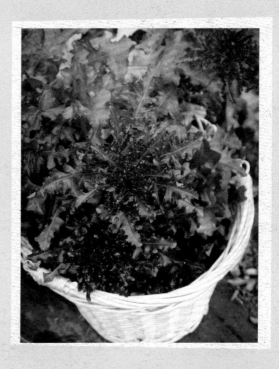

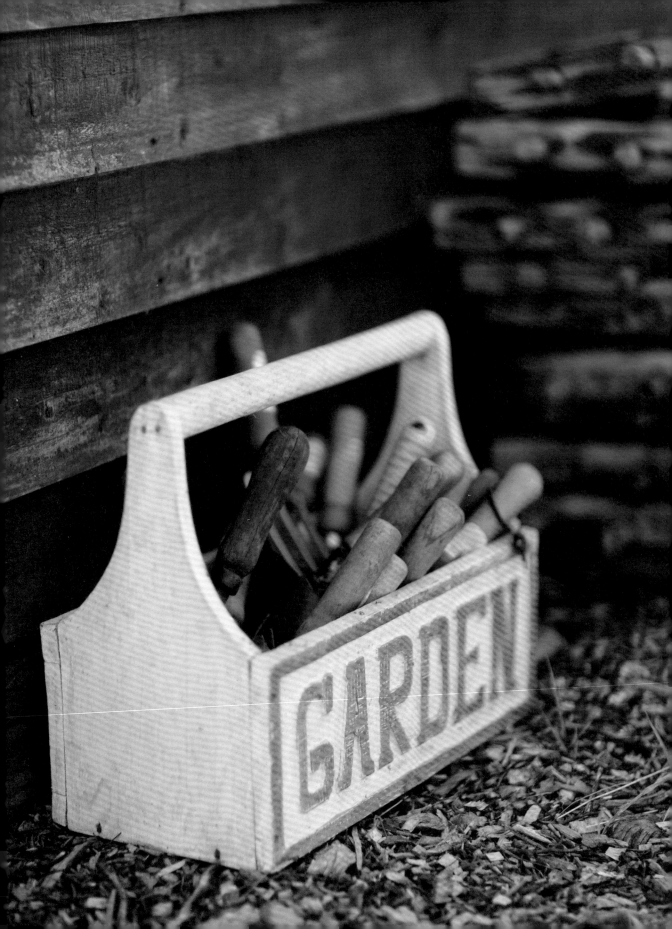

perishable crops, and in autumn and winter there is always a glut of game which can be turned into delicious pâtés and casseroles. If you buy seasonally and think creatively, you can cash in a glut of fruit or vegetables to make mountains of jams, chutneys and puddings for the price of a few bottles of vinegar, oil and spices, or a little sugar, butter and flour.

Don't forget that even a gardenless homeowner is a landowner on one level. Roadside verges, parks, canal towpaths and footpath hedges are effectively public property, so anyone can gather seasonal buckets of berries, nuts and edible fungi. Many of these are not only far superior in taste and quality to anything you can cultivate yourself, but are potentially expensive delicacies too – such as hop shoots, bilberries (myrtilles to the French) and porcini mushrooms.

Surprisingly, even keeping livestock is still an option in a very small space –

albeit not inside your home. For instance, you don't need land to be a beekeeper. Cities and towns are great foraging grounds for these industrious little insects because other people's gardens and parks are full of flowers and blossom for most of the spring and summer. As a result London now boasts hundreds of rooftop hives. The workers quietly buzz in and out, usually completely unbeknownst to the neighbours, producing hundreds of kilos of honey for very little human effort.

Once you have a bit of experience under your belt you can then branch out and try beekeeping at a distance, and you may find that you are able to produce honey with no land – or even roof – at all. Most farmers will willingly fence off a corner of one of their fields in return for free pollination of their crops. Indeed, many fruit growers will actually pay beekeepers to move hives into their orchards in spring.

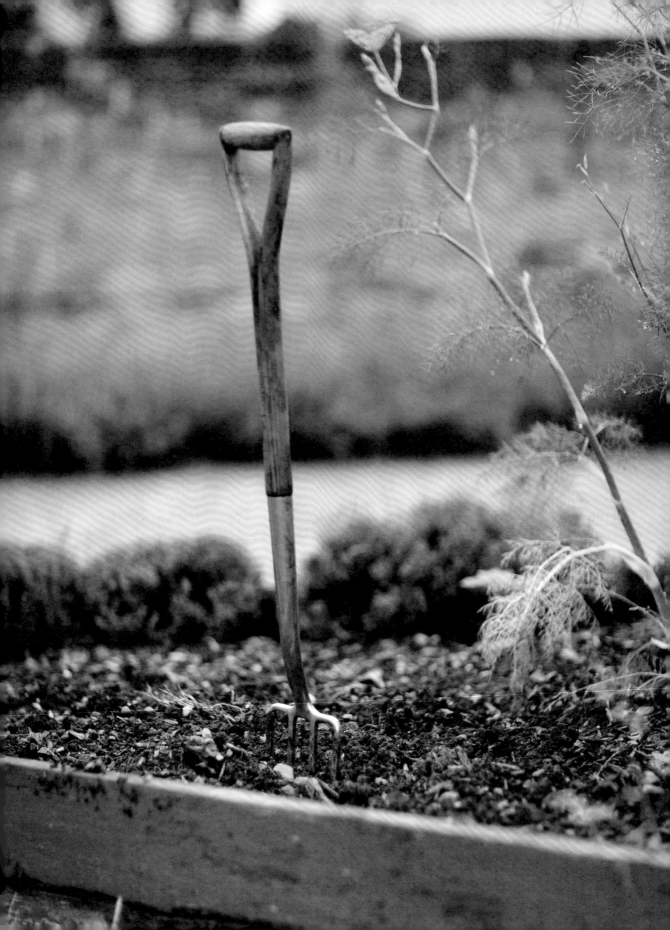

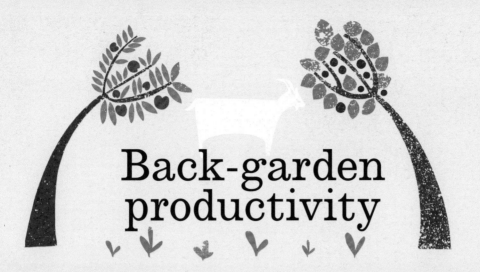

Back-garden productivity

If you're lucky enough to have a garden, your productivity has just increased significantly – with a little careful planning you can grow a great deal of food on even the smallest patio.

The 1970s sit-com, *The Good Life*, might have poked fun at the niceties of middle-class suburbia, but the truth is you can genuinely produce most of a family's food needs in a moderately sized garden. Indeed, you can do a great deal if you are imaginative, do your research into each plant or variety's requirements and target your efforts intelligently.

Among the first considerations – and this actually applies to all growing and rearing – are the local weather conditions, soil type and situation. The first two will have a huge bearing on what crops will grow well and may have implications for livestock too. The last is often overlooked, but is equally important. For example, if you have a large, south-facing wall in a sheltered garden you can grow some surprisingly delicate plants – espalier apricots and cherries, for example, or even grapes.

This also often applies to apparently soil-less patios. These may have originally been designed as suntraps for humans, but plants love the same conditions, particularly because paving stones soak up heat during the day and then slowly release it at night, rather like a sort of solar-powered night storage heater. This means tubs or raised beds situated here can be extremely productive.

Growbags, too, are good as temporary 'beds' for plants. They are cheaply available from supermarkets and garden centres and take up only a little space. You can extend the usage of these over a longer growing season, too, thereby increasing the plants' output, by covering them with a transparent plastic tent to make a 'micro-greenhouse'.

There is plenty you can do in the smallest garden, although you will need to do a bit more planning in order to

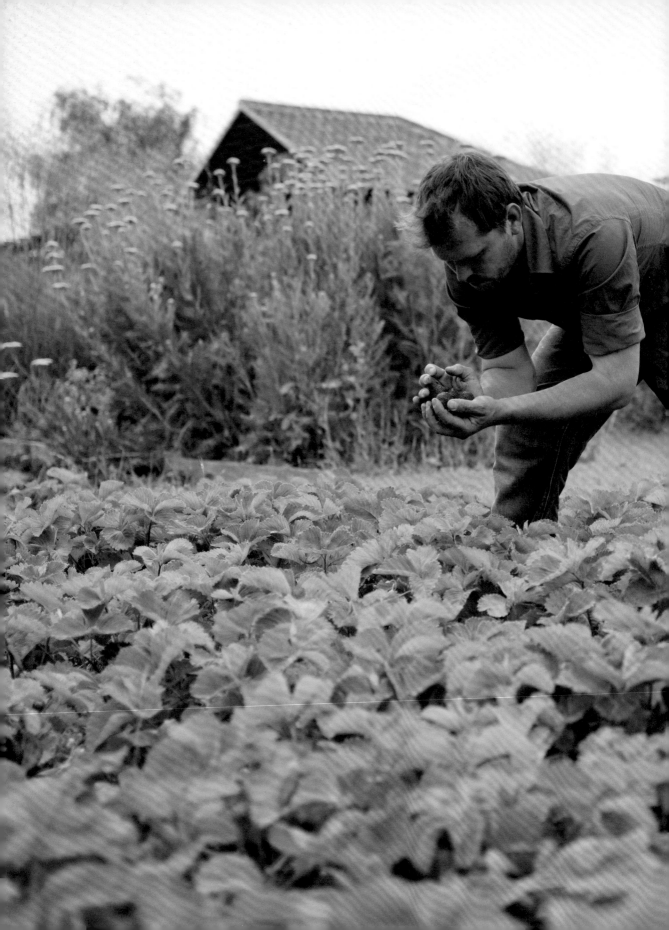

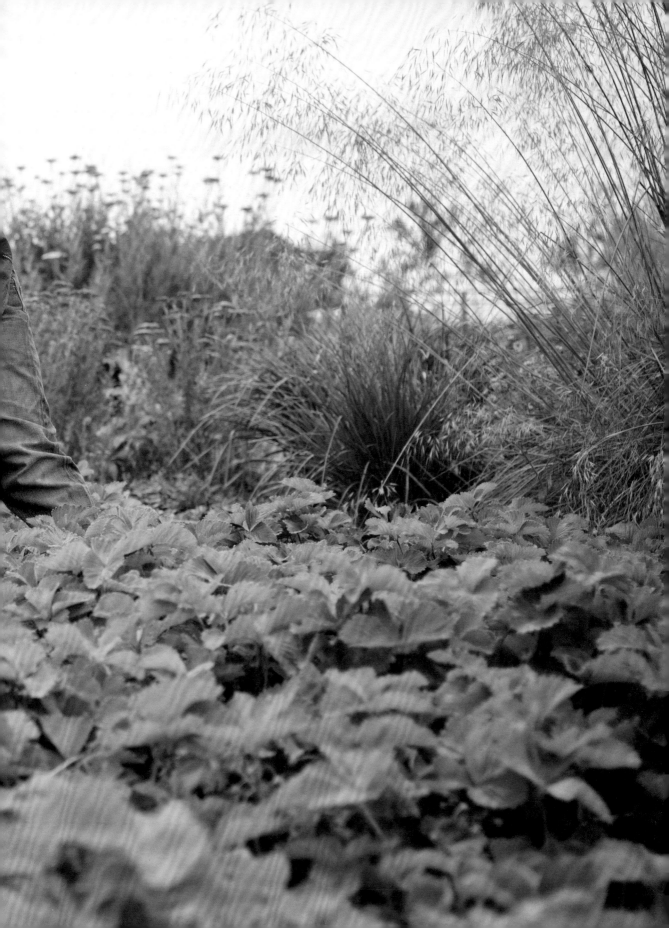

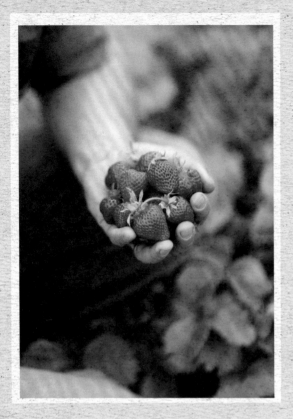

and smell problems, so there may be local restrictions on keeping such animals. Before you go out and buy animals, the best advice is to check first with your neighbours, trading standards and environmental health departments and establish if there are any objections to you keeping livestock.

Bountiful beds and borders

Vegetable beds have more modest space requirements; three or four beds (preferably raised, to increase soil temperature and ease of access) will supply enough vegetables to feed a family for most of the year, with occasional surpluses that can be sold or processed into jams, pickles and chutneys. Productive raised beds can also be made to look good or simply blend into your garden when planted up with striking vegetables such as globe artichokes, colourful chards or purple basil, thus giving you the double whammy of an attractive garden feature as well as providing delicious food.

The options become greater still if you add a moderately sized greenhouse – let alone the possibilities of a polytunnel. These will not only greatly extend the growing season of your crops but will also allow you to raise your own seedlings. By starting plants off in this way you can maximise the output from your vegetable beds, because as soon as you harvest one crop you can transplant young plants to replace them, rather than having to start

maximise your output. Potatoes will crop heavily in an old dustbin or even a strong plastic sack filled with compost, while herbs, strawberries and tomatoes thrive in tub planters. There is much to be said for these because, unlike conventional beds, they are relatively weed-free, meaning they can be very productive in a small space with very little maintenance.

It goes without saying that the bigger the garden the more flexibility you have. In larger gardens it may even be possible to keep smaller breeds of sheep, such as Soays, or perhaps goats (but these will devastate vegetable patches or flower borders unless strictly controlled). Pigs can also be just about possible, but all of these bigger creatures can cause noise from seed all over again and thereby losing precious weeks of harvesting time. As well as shortening the gaps between cropping, this 'successional planting' also keeps the soil at least partially covered and shaded all the time, preventing weed invasions and reducing your weeding work. It also allows you to have young plants ready to go into the ground as soon as the frosts have passed, meaning you can get ahead of the game because the plants will be ready to crop sooner.

Urban livestock

If you have set your heart on having an animal or two, keeping rabbits and chickens is certainly possible, even in a modest garden. These animals will live inexpensively on kitchen and garden scraps, producing eggs and meat. Also, provided their rich manure is properly rotted down (see 'composting', pp.66–7), they can provide a valuable fertiliser for your plants, reducing your expensive imports from the garden centre.

Rabbits and chickens have modest space requirements and are very happy in a movable ark with a run that you can shift across the lawn. It can be even nicer to allow the chickens to range freely, feeding on insect pests in the vegetable patch. Bantams (which are just miniature hens) are generally content to restrict themselves to creepy crawlies, but the bigger hens can develop a taste for your crops, so keep a wary eye on them. All

chickens are descended from jungle fowl, which live in family groups, so the domesticated birds are happiest in small groups of hens with one or two cockerels. The last will crow, however, which can be charming for the owner, but neighbours may be less enthusiastic in mid-summer when the noise begins at dawn.

Another downside is that both rabbits and hens are magnets for foxes. In the countryside persecution means these predators are wary and generally nocturnal, but urban foxes have lost their fear and can be remarkably bold – they are quite happy to seize your pets in broad daylight under your very nose. This means that unless you are very lucky you will have inevitable losses.

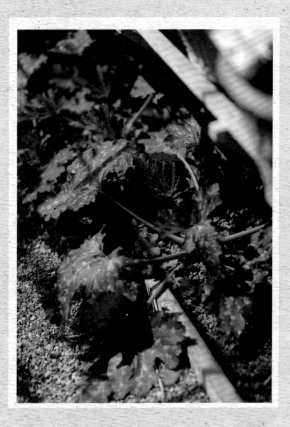

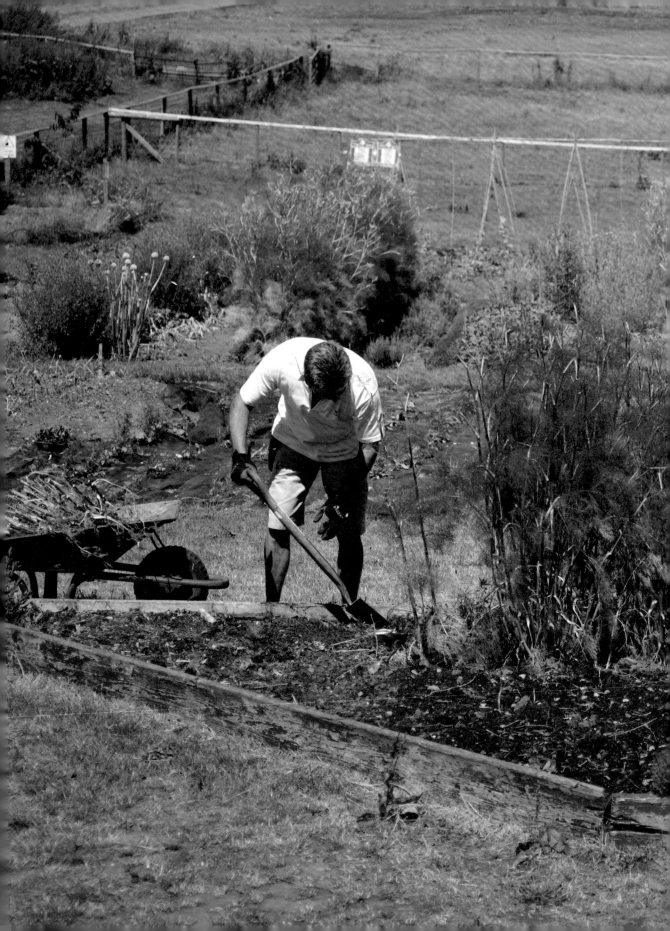

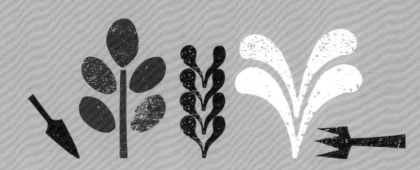

Leasing an allotment

If you don't have much space and a window box of salads and herbs just isn't satisfying your self-sufficient urges, another option is to think bigger and get an allotment.

It may be surprising to learn that councils are legally obliged to provide allotments to local residents; however, the problem is that in most areas where development land is worth a fortune (i.e. almost all cities), the demand for these lovely plots far outstrips supply and waiting lists can be several years long. If you are lucky enough to get your hands on one, this is a great way to get into food production, not least because of all the help and advice that is usually available from enthusiastic and experienced allotment neighbours.

However, this is a big step up from a couple of pots, growbags, or even raised beds; having an allotment demands commitment and plenty of your time (particularly in spring and summer), so do make sure that any plot you take on is fairly close to your home or work so you don't lose precious time getting there. Be aware, too, that most allotment committees will inspect your plot on a regular basis and you can lose it if you do not keep it weed-free and productive.

The standard full-size allotment usually measures 10 'rods' or 'poles' – 10 x 5 metres – which is big enough to grow most of the fresh vegetables a normal family would eat (in summer, at any rate). The plot offered to you might be a full or a half-size, so rent the space you know you will be able to cope with.

The price of renting an allotment can vary widely from borough to borough and depends on the size of the plot, but generally they are not expensive to lease. On the downside, however, allotment leases usually preclude you from selling any of your produce, so you should check the small print carefully if this is likely to affect your plans.

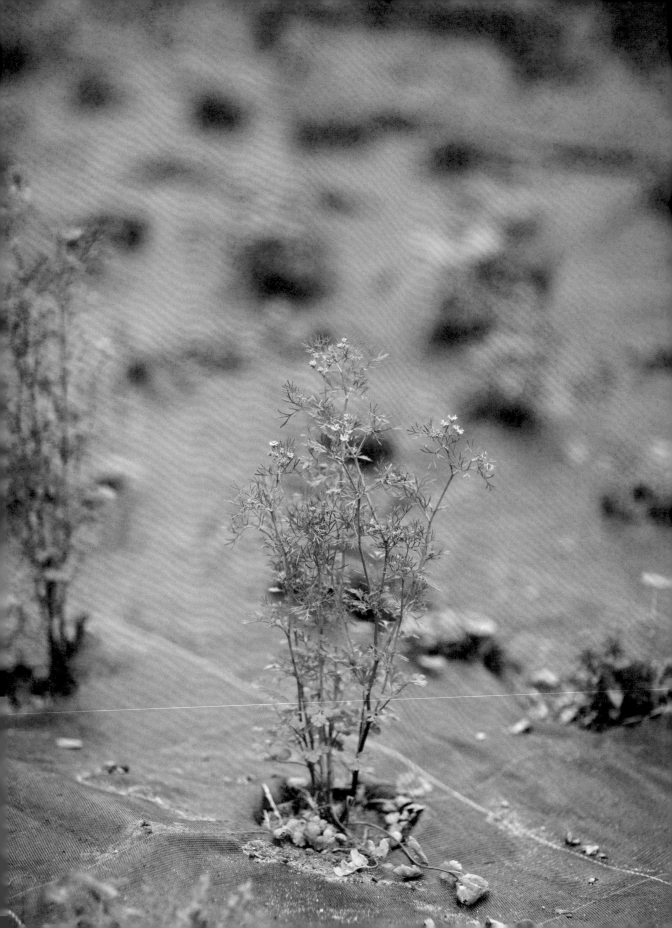

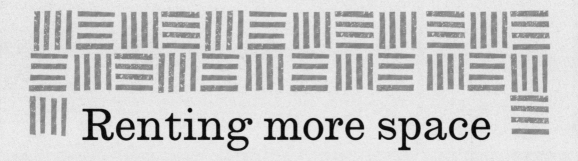

Renting more space

If turning your garden over to vegetables and livestock isn't an option and the waiting list for an allotment is too long, you might want to consider leasing more land to help you realise your productive dreams.

If you live in the country, or in more rural areas on the outskirts of towns, it might be an option to rent a field or just a portion of one. Many landowners have odd corners of land for which they have no particular use for a year or two, and while they may not want to sell these they are often amenable to leasing them out to people who will tend them and keep them in good condition, particularly if they can see it's for a worthy cause. The great advantage of such an arrangement from your point of view is that it gives you a chance to learn about your chosen produce and its potential markets without tying up large amounts of capital.

Buying a field

If you are hoping to make more of a career of your passion for homegrown or home-reared produce, you will definitely need to get your hands on a more significant amount of space. Land soars in value when it comes as part of a package with buildings, but is usually much cheaper when it is on its own: even more so if access for big farm vehicles is awkward. Unless you plan to plough your scrap of land, this may well not be a problem. Many would-be smallholders often discover that they can put their plans into operation with little more than an old four-wheel-drive or even just a wheelbarrow. One of the great benefits of buying even just a little land is that it leaves you with collateral – a clear asset against which you can borrow money to develop your business as, hopefully, it grows.

All this means that even the old railway lines, ancient scrub and rubbish-choked little quarries which are common in many areas can be feasible options. If you can't face clearing out the weeds yourself, using goats, pigs and sheep as animal groundsmen can work (many Wildlife Trusts use this as a cheap maintenance technique on their reserves).

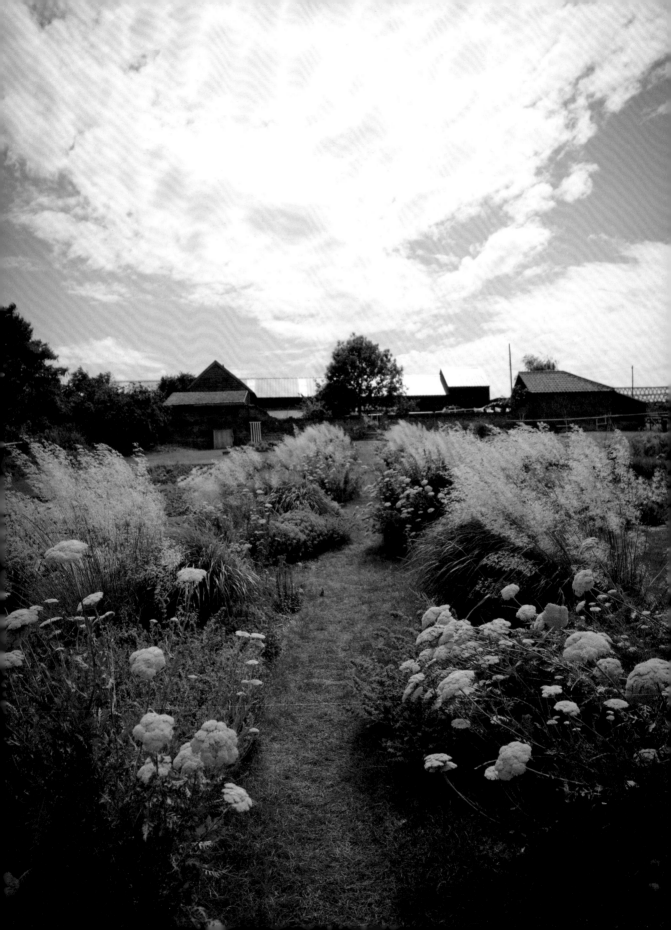

Your own farm

For many people, the ultimate dream is to buy a smallholding (by which I mean a property with two or three acres and possibly an outbuilding or two) where they can be self-sufficient or even carve out some sort of living. However, before you can turn the dream into a reality you need to make a few practical decisions.

Firstly, consider your budget. Farms can be very expensive if they are close to the big cities because these properties have the advantage of proximity to markets and often the land is of a good quality. Every year thousands of these little farms come on the market, but due to the pressure on land for development and the intensification of agriculture in many areas, the bulk of these are in the west and north. Many are very beautiful in their own right, set in spectacular scenery, and some even appear to have plenty of land. Such places are also often very affordable when compared with a cramped urban terraced house. What could be simpler than settling into a blissful existence of growing and rearing your own produce surrounded by open country, pure air and fantastic views?

The reality, of course, is much more complex. Although perfectly achievable, owning and managing a smallholding requires careful planning, research and pragmatism at the outset to turn the dream into a reality. If it were easy to earn a living from the land, British farming would not be in the state it's in now, and if there was a goldmine sitting in those fields that picture-postcard farm wouldn't be half the price of a London semi. When a lovely old building surrounded by open fields seems cheap, there is almost always a very good reason.

So, consider the land price; the value of the site is closely tied to the potential output. Near cities land values can soar to hundreds of thousands – even millions – of pounds per acre if there is a chance of development, but putting that aside, a prime arable field in Essex may be worth ten times the same area in the Highlands.

There are several factors affecting the agricultural potential of farmland. The local climate is obviously very important. Average temperatures, rainfall and even wind will affect what you can grow and rear. Some goats are quite delicate, for example, and will struggle with a Pennine winter, while pigs will turn wet ground into a quagmire and chickens don't like wind. You can get round this by providing shelter and moving them indoors in winter, but this is trickier with delicate plants (although not necessarily impossible).

So it is always important to do your research carefully and either look for a property in an area that suits your dream or buy your ideal property and then tailor your produce to suit it. If you try to do both at the same time you can easily end up hammering a square peg into a round hole.

Making the most of hill farms

Every year thousands of small hill farms come onto the market across the West Country, Wales, the Pennines and Scotland. These can seem very affordable, but there are good reasons why so many farmers can't persuade the next generation to take over the family farm. Put simply, their sons and daughters know just how tough life can be running a business on such farms and so they prefer to seek an easier, more affluent lifestyle away in the cities.

One of the most important underlying reasons for the difficulty of farming here is, quite simply, the altitude; don't forget that temperatures drop by an average of 2–3°C with every 300m of height above sea level. Put another way, moving to a farm on a moderately sized mountain is the equivalent of moving 350 miles towards the Arctic. That might not seem much, but the Dordogne is 350 miles south of London, while Gleneagles is 350 miles further north. Tomatoes, aubergines and melons thrive in the first, are possible in the second, but totally impractical in the Grampians – unless you shift your theoretical position back south with the heavy use of greenhouses and artificial heat. This means you will struggle to grow most – although not all – crops in hilly areas.

Another important factor is that in hilly areas the land is almost always poor, often with thin acidic soil, and the climate is usually harsh, battered by wind, rain and snow. Of course, grass still grows on our mountains, which is why most hilly regions in Britain are livestock rather than arable areas, but even this has its own growing requirements. Not surprisingly, the species that do best are the wild, indigenous ones that have evolved to cope with the conditions.

There's nothing wrong with turning to wild, indigenous grasses for your fodder. Indeed, it is very important that we continue to graze these grasses and herbs because many native invertebrates have highly specialised dietary and habitat requirements, and maintaining ancient

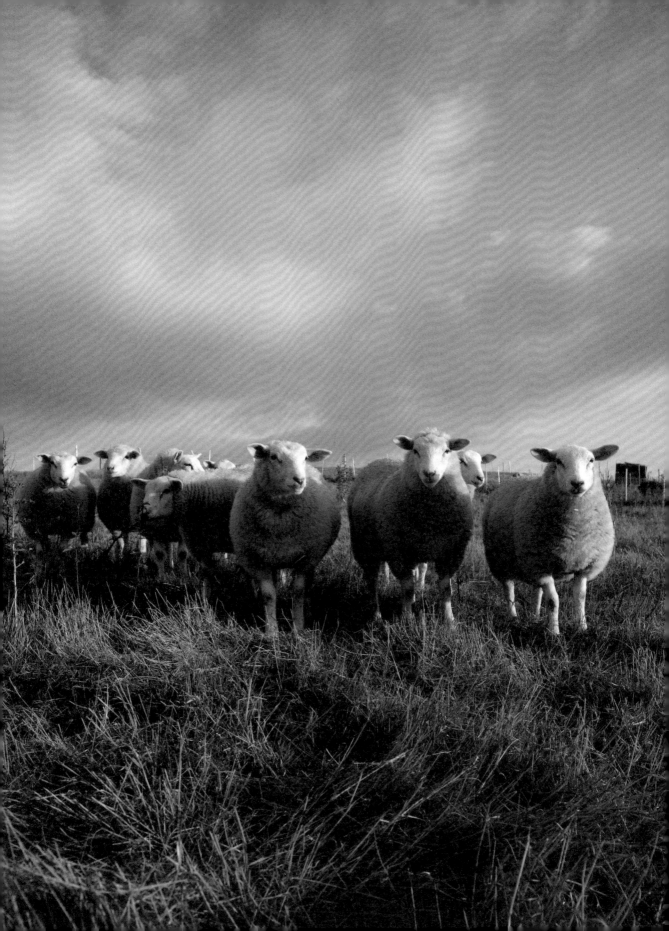

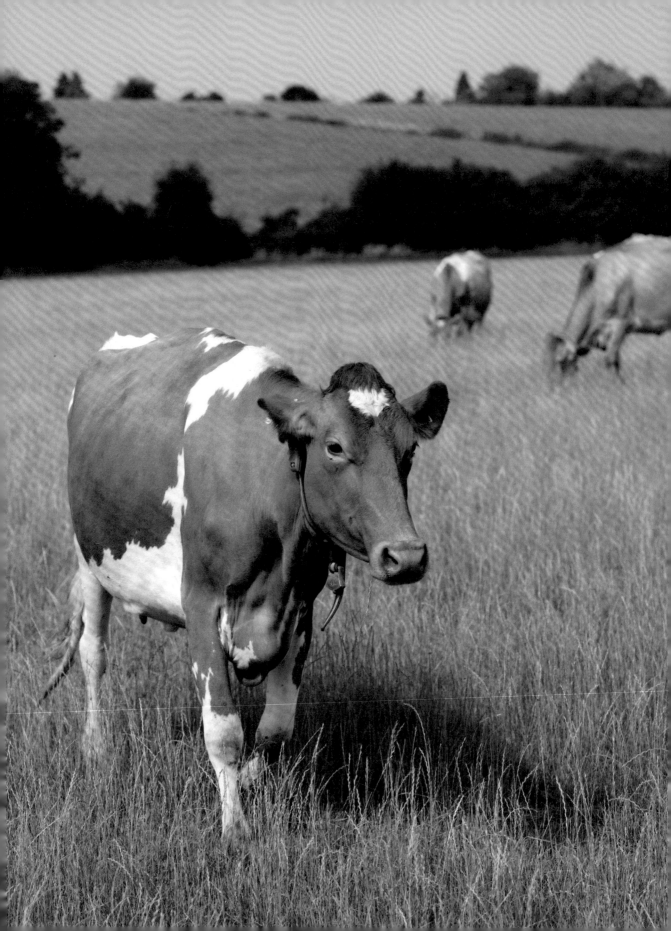

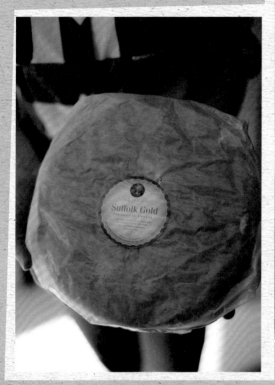

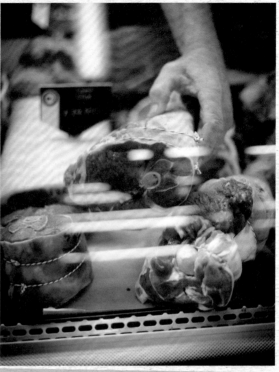

pasture is important for biodiversity. However, the farmer needs to recognise that these grasses are short of carbohydrates and nutrients. As a result, unless you buy in a lot of expensive food, stocking densities plummet with altitude, so the amount of land you need in order to make a living goes up. This means that while you can earn pocket money and have fun on a smallholding of a dozen acres, to make any sort of a living generally requires a minimum of 100 acres – and even then you will need to be imaginative and work hard. On the positive side, though, while keeping upland livestock can be labour intensive, it doesn't require a lot of expensive machinery.

One good tip for working out the most realistic possibilities for your own personal situation is to see what the neighbours are producing and the size of their holdings. Up to about 200 metres this can mean either cattle or sheep and it could also allow both meat and milk production. Above this, however, milk production (which requires lush grass or extra concentrates) becomes difficult, and above 300 metres even the hardier varieties of beef cattle start to struggle.

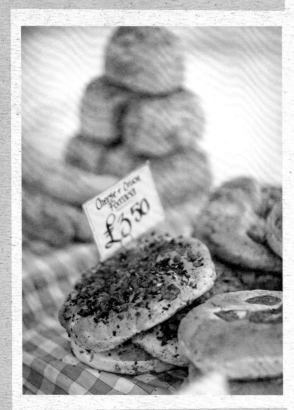

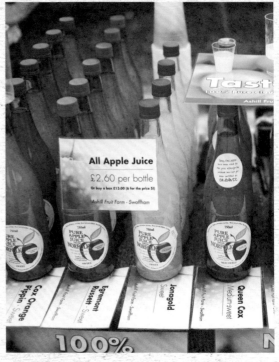

All Apple Juice
£2.60 per bottle
Or buy a box £13.00 (6 for the price 5)

Ashill Fruit Farm - Swaffham

100%

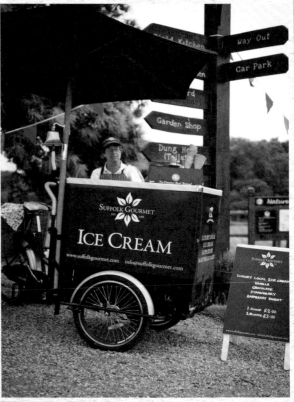

ICE CREAM

SUFFOLK GOURMET

www.suffolkgourmet.com
info@suffolkgourmet.com

Find a NICHE or an ANGLE that sets your product apart from those of the EXPERTS who have been farming the area for GENERATIONS

This means most upland farms depend on sheep, and the higher the land, the more this means the mountain breeds. These are hardier, but being smaller and having fewer lambs they are less productive.

This doesn't mean you need to slavishly copy your neighbours' examples, though: far from it. Instead, you are better off finding a niche or an angle that sets your product apart from those of the experts who have been farming the area for generations. What they do is still a good indicator of what is possible, however, and that is where you should start your search for a winning formula.

So, while it could be clear that it is most feasible to keep sheep rather than beef or to use the land for arable farming, this doesn't necessarily mean you should turn to churning out lamb. Mutton is increasingly fashionable, for example (see pp.86–7 for one man's experience in this market), but there are alternative grazers. Some of the hardier strains of goat will do well on rocky scrub, while geese can thrive on upland grass (remember many wild species fly to the Arctic Circle to breed).

Commercial farming

If you have ambitions to grow or rear for sale rather than simply for self-sufficiency, then the major issue you will need to address is where will you find your customers? Rural areas are, by definition, thinly populated, which can make it difficult to drum up sales. Suffolk is generally thought of as being fairly densely populated, but I couldn't survive on sales within the local area alone, and taking my produce out to more crowded, wealthier towns and cities takes both time and money. We certainly do go to a range of farmers' markets and food fairs across East Anglia, but it's costly to do so.

One device being used by an increasing number of producers – including me – is to get Mohammed to come to the mountain. In other words, if you need to get customers, you need to find ways of getting them to visit you. We have a range of attractions on the farm which make a visit a great family day out – nature walks, petting corners, old tractors to climb on, plenty of information, plus, of course, the farm shop and restaurant.

One way of getting people to come to your farm – and of adding value to your product – is to build in an invitation to visit your property on your labelling. If, having tasted your product, or even just having visited your website, someone then takes the time to drive a couple of hours to see your happy roaming livestock or your organic vegetable patch, they will rarely get back in their cars and go home empty-handed.

Now we're lucky to be based within easy range of millions of people, but the same idea could be applied much further afield, you just have to work that much harder to persuade customers that the journey is worth it.

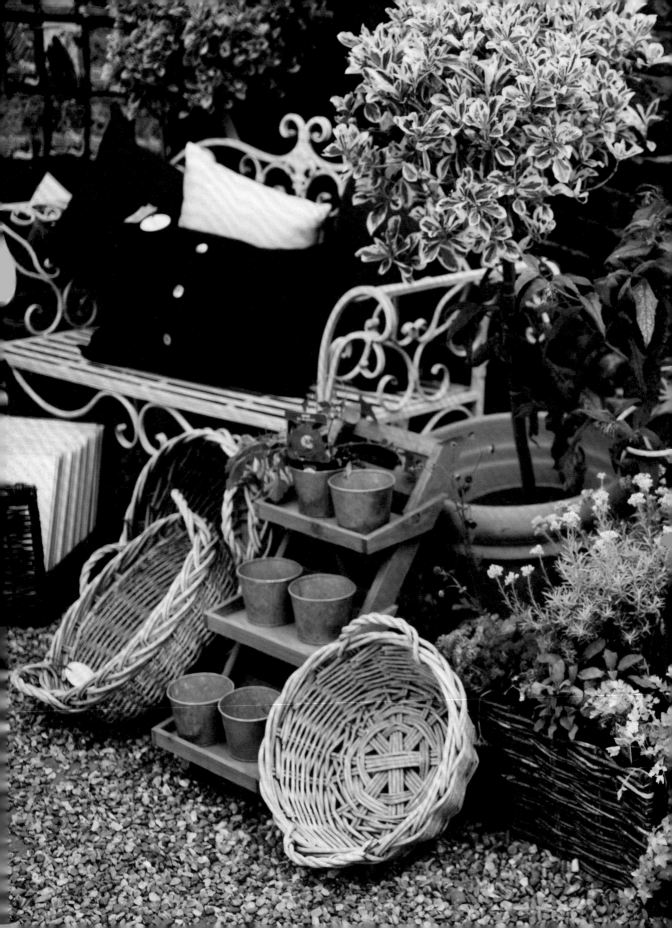

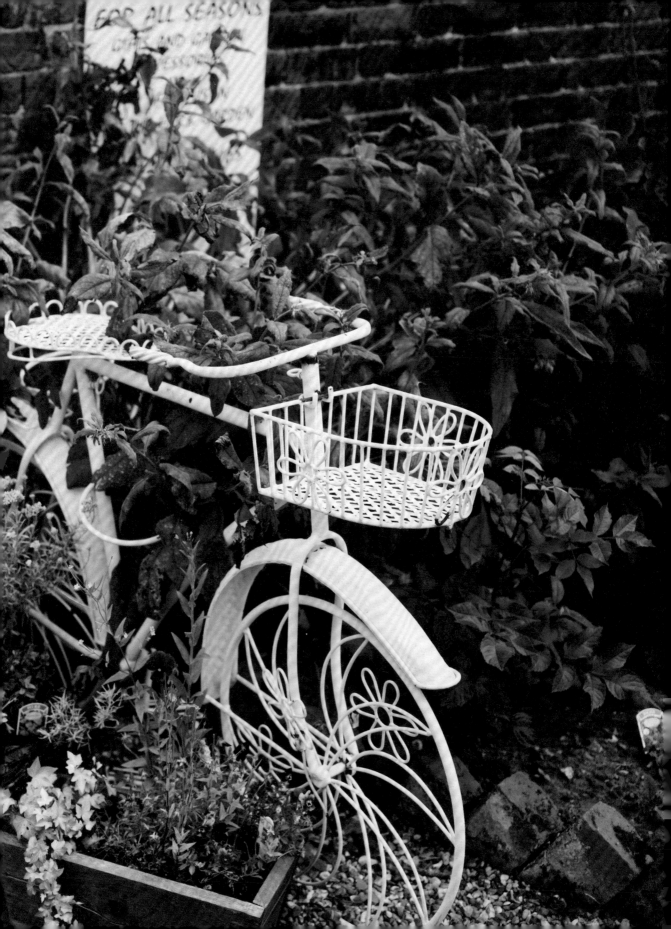

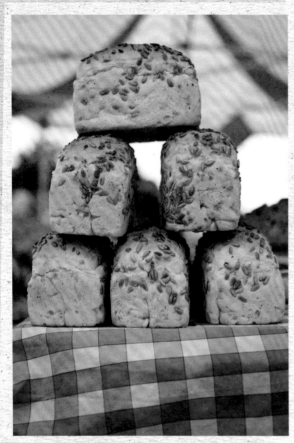

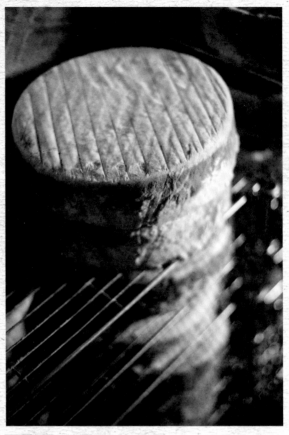

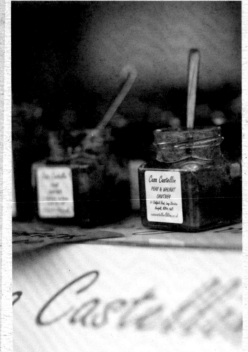

Many small producers WELCOME help... whether this means manning a VEGETABLE STALL, packing ORGANIC BOXES, BOTTLING chutneys, or WEEDING the VEGETABLE PLOT

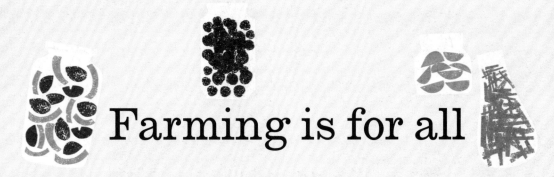

Farming is for all

If you've considered every option we've suggested so far and you simply can't get hold of enough land near you to be able to grow or keep what you want, you might need to think of other ways to produce your own food.

One solution to this dilemma is to think co-operatively; you may lack the space or time during the week to tend your crops or livestock, but other people may have the opposite problem. Many small producers welcome help at weekends, for example, whether this means manning a vegetable stall, packing organic boxes, bottling chutneys or weeding the vegetable plot. You can do this on a cash-in-hand basis, but a cashless 'produce for labour' arrangement is often better for all.

At the more unusual extreme, you might be able to find someone who rears a cow or a couple of pigs each year – producing too much for one family to consume, but not enough to sell. If you can come to an arrangement whereby you split some of the work and the bills along the way, you can divide up the final carcass between you all, having shared the effort and enjoyment of rearing your own meat for your plate.

So farming can be for all, on some scale or another, and it is possible for everyone to live the dream if you are realistic in your ideas and approach from the outset. Growing and rearing your own produce can be hard work and it is easy to spend a lot of money and get very little in return.

Nevertheless, the whole process can be hugely enjoyable, and with just a little thought and some careful planning you can grow, rear or make something that is rewarding on every level. At its simplest this might be no more than growing a handful of herbs in a window box to liven up your cooking, or a few unusual vegetables in a back garden, but more ambitious souls could aspire to producing a range of chutneys or jams from the produce from an orchard, allotment or small farm, while others could aim for egg, meat or even cheese production if they have more land.

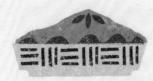

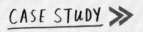

CASE STUDY »

CASE STUDY

LESLEY Wickham STARTED her 'Good Life' Dream in the 1970s In GLOUCESTERSHIRE.

Brought up with horses, Lesley's dream was simply to move her Welsh cob mare, its two-year-old and her new colt onto the four acres that came with her Forest of Dean home. 'Unfortunately, the previous owner had kept horses but had neglected the land and so it had gone "sour" for horses,' she says. 'They are selective grazers and only take the good grazing, but even so, if three mountain cobs can't get enough to eat on four acres something has gone wrong.'

So she started to branch out into other livestock to slowly improve her own land and found herself renting fields for the horses. 'In the end we were doing 30 miles a day in round trips, and it started to get wearing,' she says. The answer was to buy a 40-hectare (100-acre) mid-Wales smallholding, which they did in 1996, and with it a resident flock of speckled (mountain) sheep. These were clearly struggling and – after 18 months – they realised the problem was mineral deficiencies in the soil.

A specialist tester visited and not only gave them a detailed analysis of what was wrong, but provided a supplement to improve the land: 'I trudged back and forth scattering it like some eighteenth-century peasant sowing corn,' laughs Lesley. This solved the problem, but a succession of wet winters leached the expensive nutrients out of the land and now Lesley relies on simply providing a seaweed-based supplement for her animals to eat at will: 'They follow their natural cravings, and if they overdo it the excess just goes into the soil,' she observes.

The next great blow came with the foot-and-mouth outbreak in 2000, which completely upended the economics of farming mountain sheep. At one point

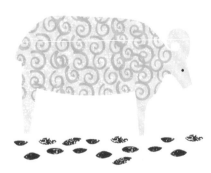

prime lambs and ewes were only worth a few pounds each – far less than the costs accrued during their production: 'For a couple of years there was no market for them, so I started to look around for new ideas,' she says. 'It was difficult, very difficult, and the answers obviously seemed to lie in other directions.'

She found these in a variety of forms, including goats, which are now central to the farm. Her 30-strong flock is her real passion. These are pedigree Boer (meat), Angora (wool) and English-based hybrids (meat). As with most livestock, the bulk of the males are destined for the table, but Lesley is generally less interested in meat production than rearing livestock for other qualities. Her pedigree Boer does are worth three or four times as much as breeding stock as they are to the abattoir. The Angoras are sheared twice a year for their wool (which she spins and uses to make knitwear, again bumping up its value as another product to sell), while the bigger genes of the English goat produce a larger carcass.

She also has 30 Dexters for beef. Their drawback is that they produce a small carcass and are slow to mature, but they are hardy, which is perfect for her farm, which nestles on the 1,000-foot contour: 'They are a wonderful breed and can live out all year, but unfortunately too many "hobby" smallholders are buying them,' she says. 'After a year or two these smallholders get bored of winter feeding and give up, selling their stock off at rock-bottom prices. This depresses the market, which is a pity because the best beef

I have ever tasted was one of my own four-year-old bulls.'

Apart from a few laying chickens which provide eggs for her own consumption, the final string to her bow is a strain of miniature sheep, Oussant. This is a rare breed which originates on an island off Brittany. They stand barely 36–40cm at the shoulder, but produce a great wool: 'It's got lovely fibres and a lot of them are black, which is ideal for spinning and knitting,' she explains. They also make wonderful pets, being perfect for a large garden or small paddock. This means that although they eat less than the mountain breeds on the surrounding hills they are worth more than their bigger versions.

Lesley has also been able to turn her fascination with wool and yarn to her advantage. She has been interested in spinning and knitting since the 1970s, but now makes a speciality out of using only her own undyed wool to make craft yarns and knitwear. Her principal lines are fleeces, carded wool, woven throws and knitwear, but the handful of lambs she kills every year for her own freezer also generate organically cured sheep skins.

This left her with the problem of how to market her produce – not easy in a low-income, sparsely populated area. The solution was to set up a co-operative with like-minded craftspeople who share the manning and costs of a co-operative shop, 'Wool and Willow', in Hay on Wye, which has been a great success. 'It is surprisingly busy throughout the year,' she laughs. 'We get customers turning up from Cardiff, Swansea and Birmingham.'

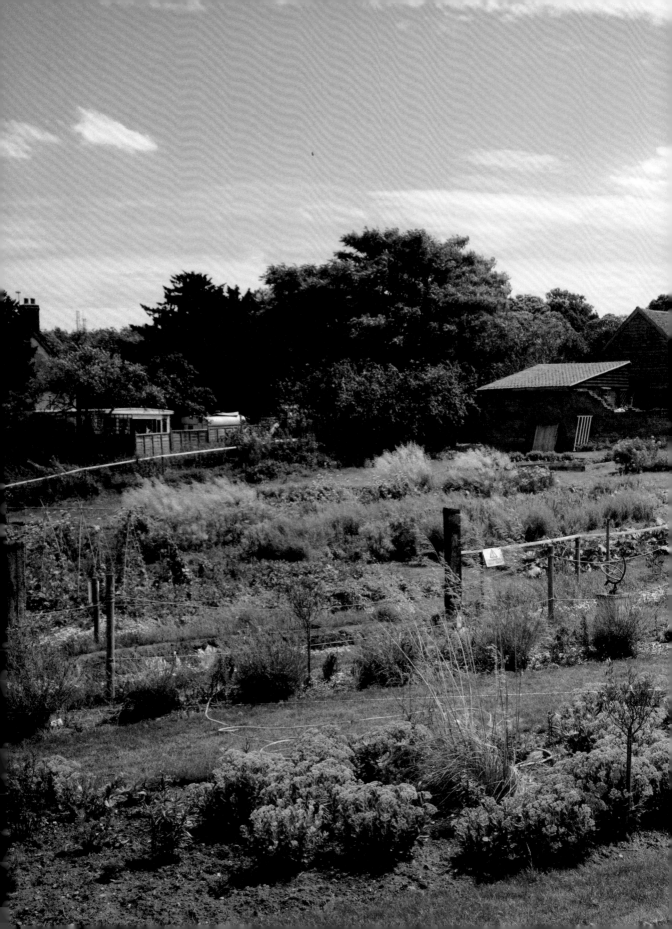

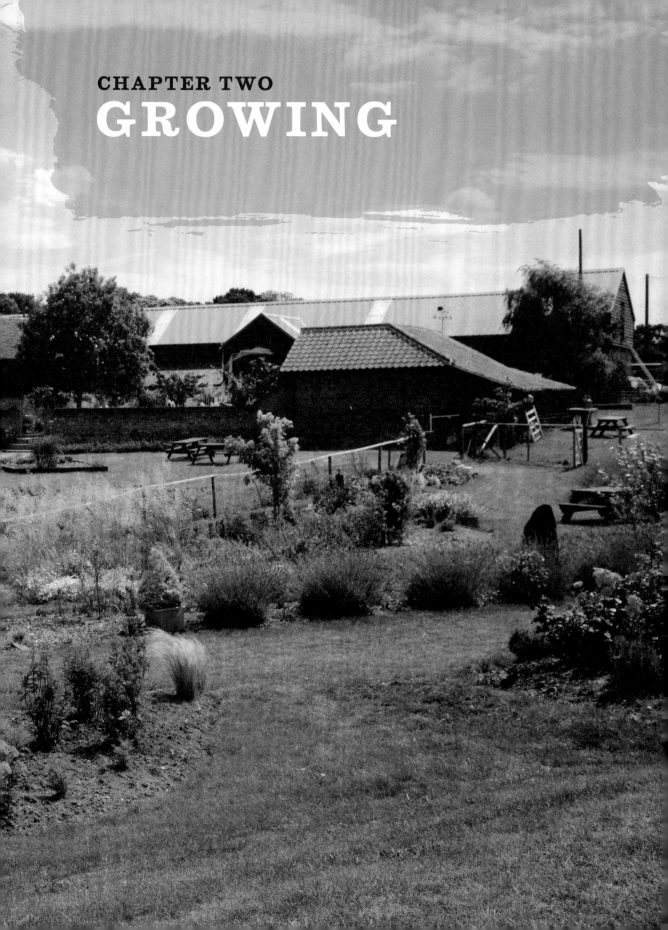

CHAPTER TWO
GROWING

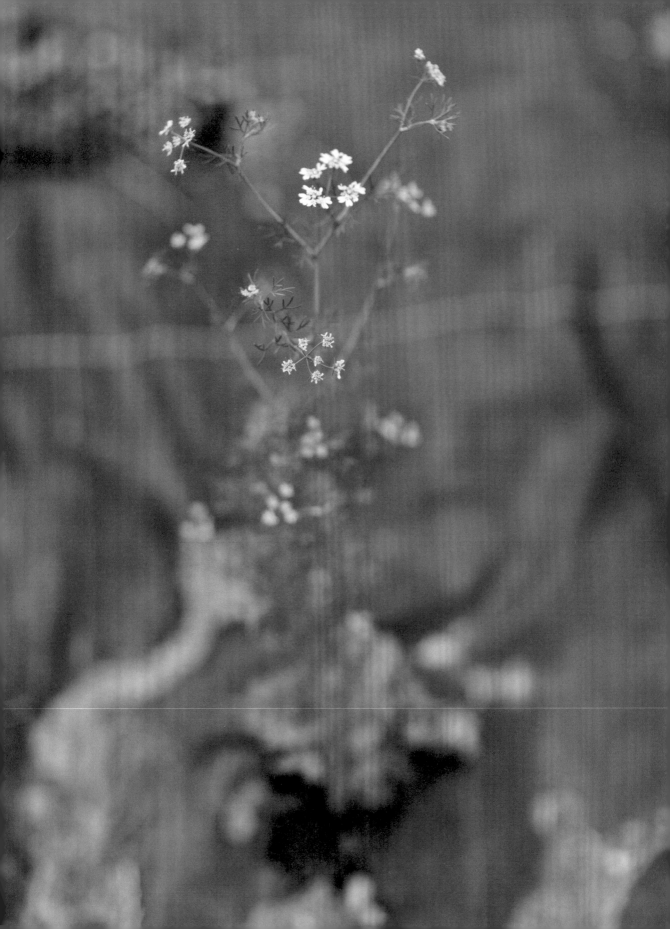

GOODIES FROM THE GROUND

THE HOME-GROWN HARVEST

Although the range and quality of vegetables and fruit available to British consumers have improved beyond all recognition over the past 20 years, there is still nothing like growing your own. Supermarkets might be able to rush crops from distant field to shelf in a just a few hours, but they can never beat the two-minute journey from garden to kitchen. Just how important this degree of freshness can be is something most people simply don't realise. With many crops it can totally transform something we take for granted – like a new potato – into the choicest delicacy.

It is also a wonderful way of hooking back into the seasons – something our modern ways of consuming encourage us to forget. Supermarkets have done a sterling job of providing steady supplies of cheap food throughout the year, and the British diet is very much the better for this, but they have also made things almost too easy. Fancy asparagus in January, or an apple in June? No problem – they are flown and shipped in from the other side of the world year-round. If you rely on your own produce, however, you learn to love nature's boom-and-bust cycles. The first June strawberry is sheer ambrosia. For the next month you gorge yourself on them until, by the end of July, you have had quite enough to last without for ten months (apart, that is, from the jars of bottled produce on the larder shelf).

It also makes you appreciate the weather more and you will find yourself glued to the forecast, listening carefully for those 'windows' when seeds are best sown or crops harvested. Most people dislike summer rain, but as a gardener you welcome a good June downpour, knowing it is only going to boost yields. Even frost and snow have their benefits, helping to suppress pests and diseases (they even improve the flavour of some crops such as parsnips).

We are actually extremely lucky to live in a country with such a comparatively mild and damp climate. If you are really determined, you can grow almost anything here – it is amazing what you can coax out of a greenhouse or polytunnel (Victorian gardeners even managed to produce pineapples in the Highlands). Of course, in practice there are many vegetables that are beyond our reach, but this is more than made up for by the thousands of seed varieties which are available from specialist suppliers. This means you can grow more exotic varieties than you will find in even the biggest superstore; from countless chillies to scores of squashes.

Growing your own is also the cheapest method of producing your own food. Unlike livestock, the set-up costs are minimal; there's no housing, vet's bills or pedigree stock to bear in mind. If you are a window-box gardener all you need is a packet of seeds and some compost, and even at the garden or allotment level the only equipment you really need is a wheelbarrow, spade, fork, hoe and watering can. Of course, you can spend a great deal on rotovators, brushcutters, greenhouses and so on, but it's not essential – certainly not to begin with.

Things get a little more complicated if you are growing to sell, but there is still much less paperwork with plants than with animals. Probably the biggest headache comes with organic registration, which requires you to keep records and sign declarations that you've only used acceptable fertilisers and forms of pest control, for example. This approach can also be fairly expensive, but the cost and effort could well be worthwhile if you can sell your produce at a decent profit.

You will almost certainly have regular gluts of crops when your plot produces far more food in a short space of time than you can cope with. Turning this into jams, chutneys or wines is the obvious solution, and it can be great fun: there is nothing to beat opening a jar of your own herb oil in midwinter and breathing in the aroma as you do so – out comes the pure scent of summer, full of the memories of heat and plenty in the garden.

Processing for sale can be a little more complicated. For a start it often involves extra work and cost. Again, because plants have fewer hygiene implications than meat or dairy, this is much less onerous, but you will still have to comply with basic food packaging and labelling regulations. Also, even moderate quantities of, say, jam or bread may quickly be beyond the average kitchen's capacity. In this case, some areas have processing units you can rent for a day or two. It is also often possible to negotiate the loan of a pub or hotel kitchen for a few hours to deal with batches too big for your own kitchen – and if you are lucky you may even be able to negotiate a cashless deal where you pay for this in produce.

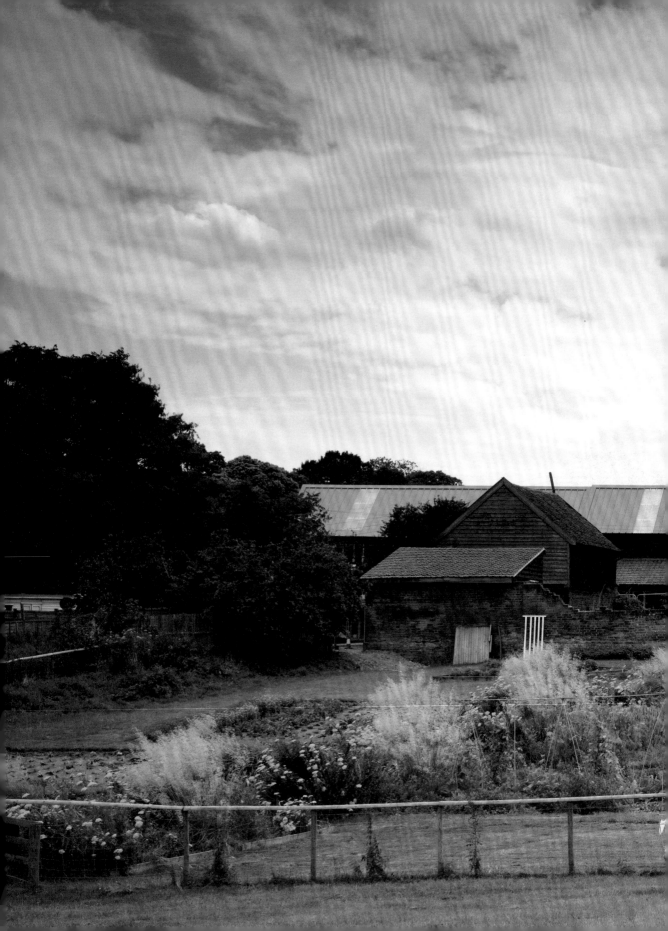

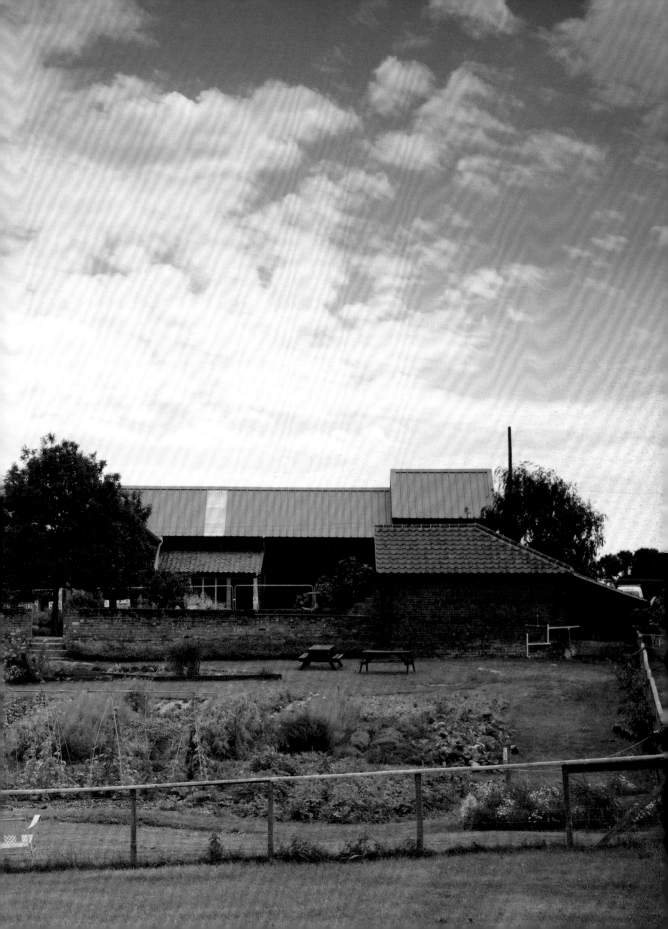

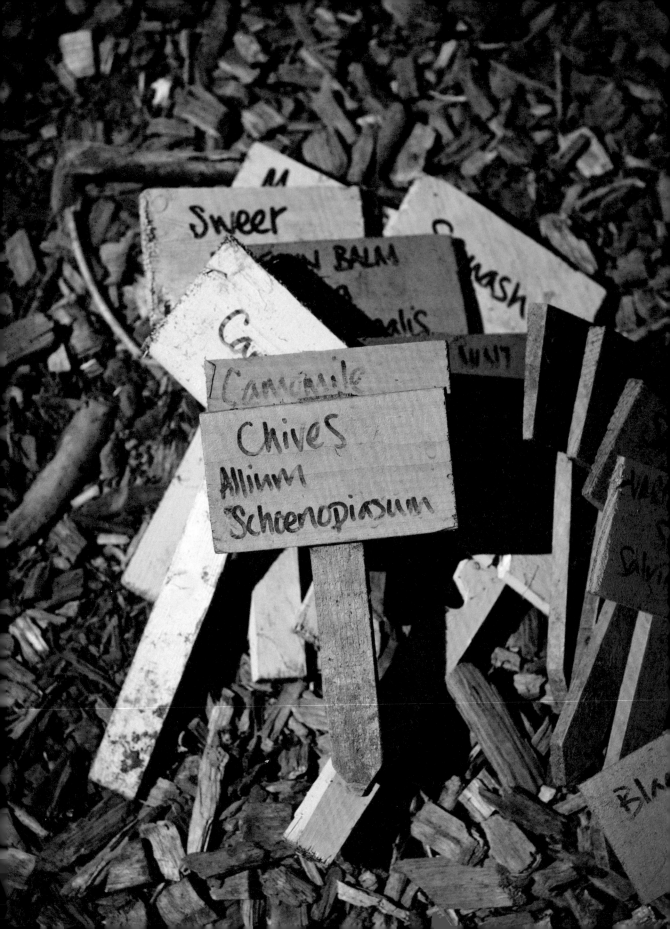

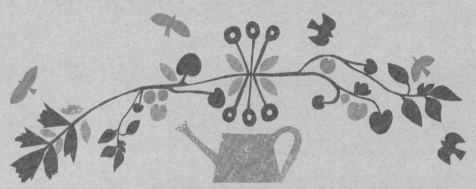

Getting started

Perhaps the most important consideration before you plan what to grow is the location of your land. Assuming you are wanting to grow something in your existing home, garden or allotment, its size, situation and aspect are critical factors in what you can grow and how well you can grow it.

The question of how much soil you have to work with speaks for itself, but its structure and quality are just as important in deciding what you can grow. Less obvious are considerations like shade, and the plot's alignment in relation to the sun is easy to overlook. Simply put, a small north-facing garden shaded by a large wall will struggle to produce many delicate plants, but the same size plot on the other side of the wall – i.e. south-facing – could burst with grapes, cherries and peaches.

It is also important to think ahead – even a lovely spot basking in the warmth of the summer sun can turn into a cold, harsh, frost pocket in winter and so you may need to bring delicate plants inside. If you can't do this because you don't have the space for a greenhouse or a polytunnel, it's not worth growing the more sensitive crops.

If you are working above ground level, say on a balcony, roof or even a window box or hanging basket, then you will also need to take your neighbours into account. You don't need to be a health and safety inspector to work out that even a small flower pot falling a few metres onto a passer-by can do a great deal of damage.

Finally, you need to consider ease of access to and within your plot. You will need to be able to work in the space, and this will include moving heavy materials such as water and compost around it. On a balcony you probably only need a watering can and a bucket, but even a small garden will most likely require a wheelbarrow and possibly hose pipe if you aren't to do serious damage to your back.

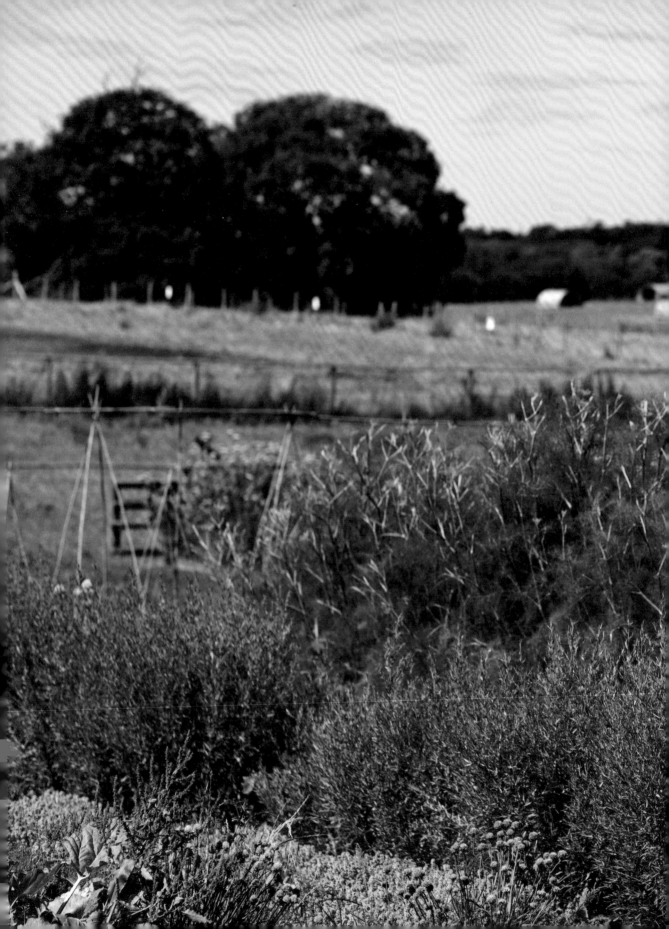

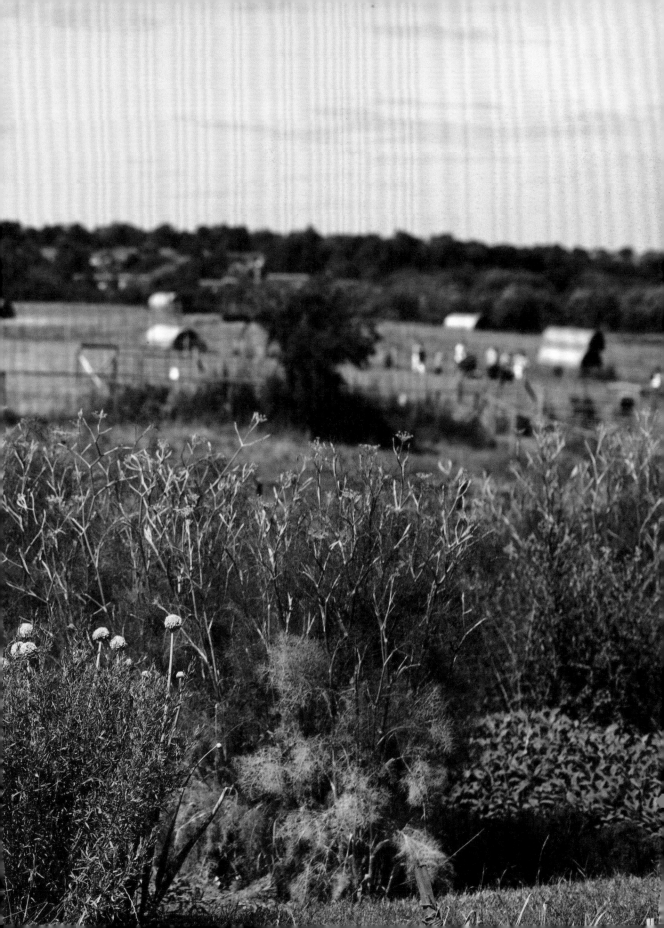

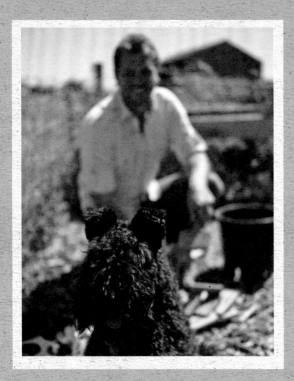

Assess what you've got

Most of the regular vegetables that you will probably consider sowing will grow almost anywhere, but the type of soil you have is also a significant factor in the success of a crop and the size of its yield.

Heavy clay soils can take time to warm up in spring, so they might not be suitable for early or delicate crops, while later on in the year they are good at retaining moisture, so plants won't need as much watering in hot dry weather. At the other extreme come the readily draining sandy soils; these are great for early crops, but nutrients tend to trickle out of them and in summer watering is usually necessary. The ideal is loam, which is somewhere between the two.

Your soil type will also affect the best choice of vegetables for your patch – for example, long thin root crops tend to grow best in light sandy soils. This doesn't mean you need to rule out carrots or parsnips on clay, however, just that you might need to cultivate shorter, rounder varieties.

You should also test your soil's acidity or alkalinity because this can have a bearing on which crops will grow best. As most people will remember from school science lessons, this is measured on a pH scale of 0–14, with 7 being neutral (the lower end of the scale is acid; the higher is alkaline). Testing is easily done at home with a cheap kit. The overall ideal is slightly acid (although some diseases, such as club root, are deterred by alkaline conditions).

You aren't necessarily completely stuck with the local conditions, though. The simplest way to deal with problem soils is to build raised beds; this effectively breaks the ground down into manageable parcels which makes it easier to alter their pH one way or the other by adding powdered limestone to reduce acidity or sulphur to make conditions less alkaline. In heavy clay areas, lifting the growing medium away from the cold waterlogged subsoil makes the soil warmer and improves its drainage. Raising the level of beds also makes access easier for routine jobs like sowing, weeding and harvesting. The downsides of raised beds are the extra expense and permanence of these constructions – and it can make it difficult or even impossible to use machinery, which can be a significant problem in even a moderate-sized garden.

Almost all soils benefit from the addition of loads of organic matter such as well-rotted manure or compost. This greatly improves nutrient levels and moisture retention. On the other hand, some crops, notably thin root crops, fare best in soils which haven't been manured too recently. In general, however, you will need to add nutrients regularly to your plot, if only to replace those you are taking out in the crops you harvest.

What to grow?

If you are only interested in growing for your own use, much the most important consideration when deciding what to grow is to sow produce that you like. Thus you might specialise in a particular herb or chilli variety whose heat is perfect for your tastes. If this is your first foray into gardening, you should take ease of growing into account, too. However, some plants require a lot more attention than others, which will grow regardless of how badly you neglect them. There's no encouragement like success, particularly at the outset, so it's probably best to avoid crops like asparagus which need a carefully prepared bed, constant weeding, and take a couple of seasons to start cropping. On the other hand, if you plant courgettes or runner beans it's hard not to have a ridiculous surplus.

On that note, one idea – particularly for the beginner or allotment holder – is to co-operate. Crop rotation and enjoyment will probably dictate that you want to grow a good variety of produce, but it is easy to get carried away. Rather than planting a little of everything, it can be sensible to sit down with one or two friends and agree a planting regime where each of you specialises in, say, a dozen vegetables. You can then each share your surplus with your friends – or if you produce enough, you could even set up your own small organic box scheme.

On the same lines, forward planning is very important generally – particularly if space is at a premium. Good crop rotation not only maximises yields, but by keeping the ground covered you help suppress weeds which will compete with your crops for nutrients and water. This isn't difficult to do, but it's well worth sitting down early in the New Year to plan the forthcoming growing season (in fact, when the weather is at its worst and the days are at their shortest, it's a good way to lift your spirits).

Many plants – such as broad beans and garlic – will actually perform better if planted in autumn or winter. Others that have long growing seasons, such as tomatoes and chillies, can be started off in a greenhouse or on a windowsill early in the season to give them a flying start. As you harvest the last of your winter cabbages, kale and purple sprouting broccoli, you can plug the gaps immediately with rows of hardier plants that don't mind a touch of frost – say, carrots, parsnips and peas – slowly trickling in more sensitive crops. Potatoes, for example, are traditionally planted at the Easter weekend when, while frost is still a risk, the germinating shoots will still be protected by the soil for another few weeks.

CLEVER COMPOSTING

Unfortunately most people's experience of composting is limited to the slimy pile of smelly grass clippings at the end of the garden, but it is actually relatively easy to make wonderful soil conditioners and fertilisers. The basic rule is to have a good mix of materials to provide the micro-organisms and worms which perform the task with all the nutrients they need.

Composting is also an important way to improve your crops because it injects vital nitrogen, phosphates, potassium, trace elements and humus into the soil. Creating a good, rich growing medium is one of the most important ways you can lift the taste and quality of your produce above their commercial equivalents. Most of these are grown with the help of artificial fertilisers in relatively inert soil (or even hydroponically in vast greenhouses).

This is also probably the most valuable form of recycling. The detritus from our kitchens and gardens accounts for 35 per cent of everything we throw away by volume, and every tonne of food consumes at least the same in CO_2 emissions thanks to fertilisers, transport and packaging. It is also by far the worst thing to go into landfill, where it rots to give off methane (20 times more powerful as a greenhouse gas than CO_2) and polluting leachates which can contaminate water courses.

A kitchen will always generate some scraps and a working garden will create far more; the important thing is to think of it not as rubbish but as a valuable resource. Many councils now offer composting schemes, but why give away something so precious? Anything the chickens won't eat can easily be turned into a rich garden fertiliser, which reduces the need to buy potentially environmentally damaging peat. There are three basic composting methods which are all suitable for gardening on a relatively small scale.

✔ TIME-SAVING TUMBLING

A modern device which works well on a small scale is a rotating bin. These are about the size of a conventional dustbin or water butt, but mounted in the middle on a spindle. Waste is fed in through a hatch and the bin is given a couple of spins to aerate the contents and make sure everything spends time in the hot centre of the pile. It is the equivalent of forking a conventional pile, but with none of the sweat, and it speeds up the process immensely. In optimum summer conditions it can take as little as a fortnight from the addition of the last material, but obviously you will need to do something with the waste you generate between adding this and emptying the bin. A second tumbler is one option, or use a model which has two compartments.

✔ GO TRADITIONAL

The traditional compost heap relies on bacteria breaking down organic material while generating enough heat to kill weed seeds, but not enough to shut everything down. This requires a mix of nitrogen and carbon, humidity and warmth. This is usually done in a large walled container, full of layers of carbon-rich 'brown' material (e.g. twigs or cardboard) with nitrogen-rich 'green' (e.g. grass clippings or kitchen waste). The former rots slowly, but keeps the pile aerated, the second generates the heat. Some manure is good, and urine is even better because it activates the pile (the human version is supposed to contain hormones which boost rooting in cuttings). Avoid cat and dog faeces because they can contain pathogens, and meat scraps can attract rats.

A good compost heap generates enough heat to kill weeds and keep the process rocketing along, but small-scale composting (particularly in winter) rarely gets hot enough. The solution is to add as much as possible at a time, use activators and insulate (for example, put old carpet over the top). Turning the heap also helps, but this can be back-breaking. In theory the composting process takes four to five weeks, but in practice this is rare on a household scale, particularly in winter. Patience and more than one bin may be the answer.

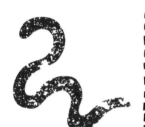

✔ WIGGLY WORM FARM

This is the most compact way in which to turn organic matter into compost. This relies not on micro-organisms and heat to break the waste down, but on hundreds of little 'brandling' worms. Once established, these are wonderfully efficient at munching their way through rubbish, turning it quickly into nutrient-rich castings. These are 11 times richer in potash, with seven times as much phosphorus, five times the nitrate and three times the exchangeable magnesium as a normal soil. As a result gardeners tend to use them as a fertiliser rather than a soil conditioner.

To start your own worm bin, take an old dustbin or wooden box, punch holes in the base and stand it on bricks for drainage (a tight-fitting lid will deter pests like foxes and rats). Put 20cm of composted bark (peat is too acidic) in the bottom and add a cup of brandlings (the small red worms you find in compost heaps, or you can buy them as bait from fishing shops). Top with a layer of kitchen waste and cover. Leave undisturbed until the worms appear on the surface, then add more material.

Once the bin is full, remove the top few inches containing the worms and remove the 'black gold'. You can improve on this basic design by collecting the juices dribbling out of the bottom (dilute this 10:1 with water for use as a liquid feed) or by adding a riddle system to sift the casts from the bottom of the heap without disturbing the occupants. For an easier life you can buy a 'Can o' Worms' – which is a stack of sieves that are small and hygienic enough to fit in most kitchens and allow compost and liquid to be removed with minimal fuss and mess.

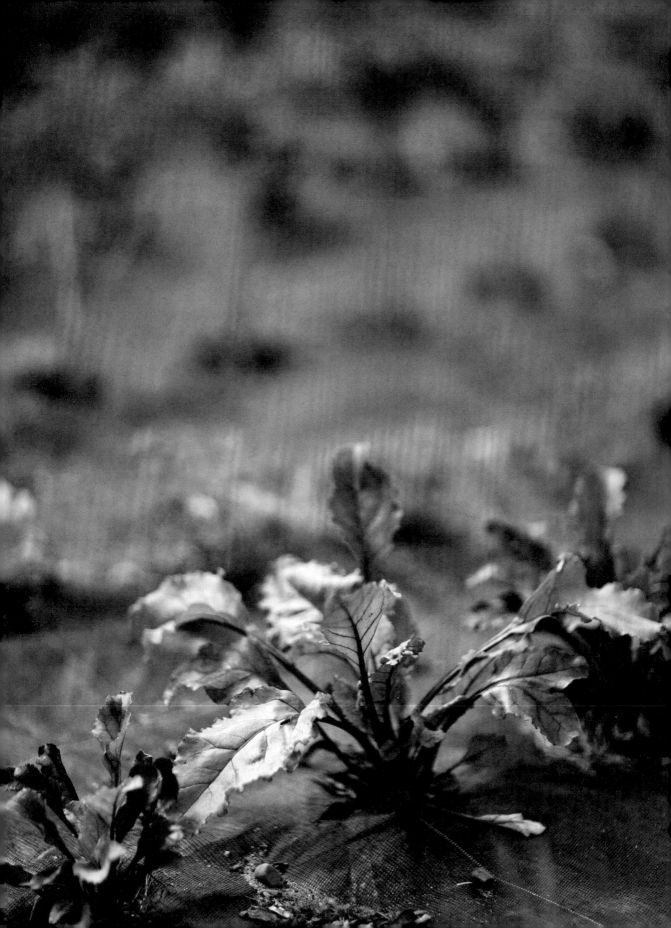

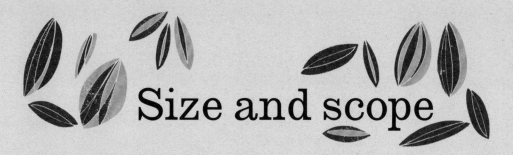

Size and scope

One of the perils of growing on any scale is that it is easy to get carried away by your own enthusiasm. So stop, think, and really plan your plot for maximum productivity and minimum wastage.

Even if you buy only one packet of seeds, if you plant them all and you live in a small flat you will be completely overwhelmed by the results. This goes all the way up the chain, of course, and I would say that the more land you have, the more important it is to stick to your plan and try to rein yourself in at the beginning of each growing season.

Small scale

You can grow plants in even the smallest upstairs flat. All you need for a steady supply of sprouting seeds or fresh mushrooms is a dark cupboard, or if you have sills, a couple of window boxes or a few flowerpots can supply most of the fresh herbs you will need in daily cooking. If you have a flat roof or balcony, strawberries, tomatoes and even potatoes become possible. You could even train

beans, peas or outdoor cucumbers up balcony railings (although you might need to tie netting to the back to give the plants something to cling to).

Of course, lack of space means you don't have the luxury of being able to leave areas empty. You will need to plan carefully what you can grow and where if you are to make the most of what you have. Herbs are the most compact way of making the biggest difference to your cooking; just a few leaves from a plant growing on a windowsill will instantly lift a dish.

Quick-growing plants play an important part in a small plot. Most salad crops take just a few weeks from sowing to harvesting. Some lettuces and leaves are designed to be 'cut-and-come-again' crops – in other words, new shoots will spring up from the stump. Others, such as beetroot, can be selectively pruned for tender young leaves while they develop their swollen roots beneath the soil. It is also often possible to grow speedy crops alongside slower varieties; thus you can plant salad leaves in the same growbags as your tomatoes. You get the first crop while it is still too cold for the delicate tomatoes to go outside and another after they have been planted out but are still too short to stifle smaller plants by hogging all the available light and nutrients.

Another important way of making the most of your available space is to use the best possible compost you can find – and don't skimp on a decent fertiliser either. Conventional growbags are all very well, but even if you can cope with the fact that most are peat-based, this is what commercial growers use and so they produce conventional-tasting plants. I've done taste tests on cherry tomatoes, planting one set in a growbag and the other in homemade organic compost which had been enriched with well-rotted chicken manure mixed with wood shavings. You would be amazed how different exactly the same variety, grown in the same greenhouse at the same time, can taste.

When space is at a premium, it is also important to be very choosy when picking varieties. Potatoes and tomatoes are relatively greedy for space and are cheap to buy in the shops, so if you are set on growing them – perhaps in a bag, bin or growbag on a balcony – it is best to make the most of your effort by planting something that rarely appears on shop shelves. For example, most retailers worry about waste so they tend to source soft fruit with the longest possible shelf life, rather than for maximum taste. With potatoes this could be an unusual salad or new variety, while with tomatoes it could be a type of tumbling yellow cherries. Similarly, if you are sprouting seeds, try to produce something a little quirky that you can't get hold of easily – perhaps cumin or a seed mix rather than the rather more familiar mung beans or alfalfa.

Obviously the same thing goes for herbs. Almost all the basil sold in this country is the green Italian or Genovese type. There is nothing wrong with it – it's one of my favourite herbs – but if I only had space for two or three plants I would go for a Thai, Greek or purple variety to give my food that extra bit of lift and colour.

Garden and allotment

The more space you have, the easier life becomes. You now have the luxury of putting out bigger plants and growing bulkier crops. For example, courgette plants will spread out too much to be practical on a balcony, but just one or two plants will provide everything you will need for your personal use. Another great quality is their flowers; these are delicious dipped in a delicate tempura batter and deep fried. Better still, because they have such a short shelf life they are genuinely unique: you just can't buy them.

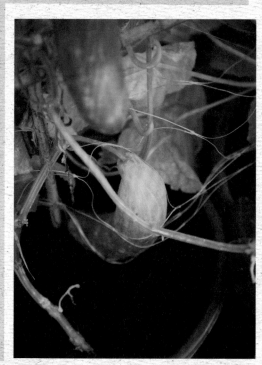

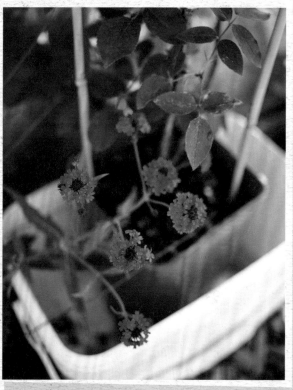

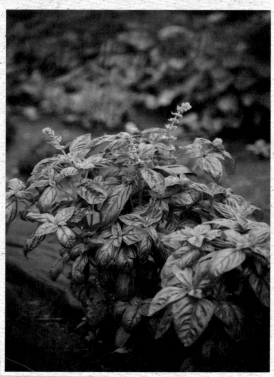

A couple of WINDOW BOXES or a few flower POTs can SUPPLY MOST of the FRESH HERBS and SALAD you will NEED in DAILY COOKING

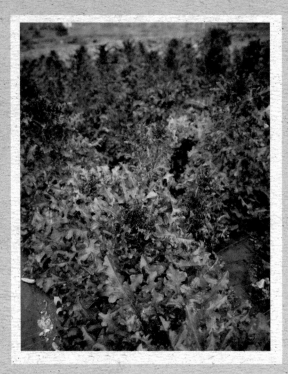

In many gardens, however, space is still a problem – particularly if you want it to be both an attractive place to relax and a productive space. There are plenty of ways to multi-task, however. For example, many vegetables are productive as well as aesthetically pleasing. A varied row of lettuces with different textures and colours – say endive, oak leaf, lollo rosso and radicchio – makes a wonderful addition to the front of a border. Also, don't forget many flowers are edible too. We don't eat many of them in this country, but calendula and nasturtiums make colourful additions to a salad while heart's-ease flowers can be frozen in ice cubes to make an attractive addition to a well-earned gin and tonic as the sun goes down.

Globe artichokes are another one of my favourites. These are ridiculously easy to grow and extremely pest-resistant. Although they are eaten in huge numbers on the Continent (Brittany is a traditional growing area, which shows that they should do well here too), as a nation we have never been so keen on them, so they feature infrequently on shop shelves – and when they do they are generally over-priced. They take up a fair amount of space, spreading to well over a metre high and the same across, but they are very ornamental, with lovely silvery foliage from the delicious flower buds that appear in high summer.

Beans are one of the most productive vegetables in terms of yield per square metre. Just one or two 'wigwams' of runner beans will supply the needs of most families. Broad beans are really worthwhile, not least because they are tough and are one of the first crops you can harvest in spring – especially if you choose one of the autumn-planting varieties. Better still, by keeping plants in the soil you help to suppress weeds and after you have finished harvesting you can clear them out completely, creating space for more delicate plants after the danger of frost has vanished.

In bigger gardens or allotments there are naturally other possibilities too. For example, you could have space for maincrop potatoes. These may be cheap to buy, but this is in large part because they are relatively trouble-free, with blight being the biggest threat (in which case you will have to intervene, but there are perfectly acceptable organic sprays, or you can buy blight-resistant varieties).

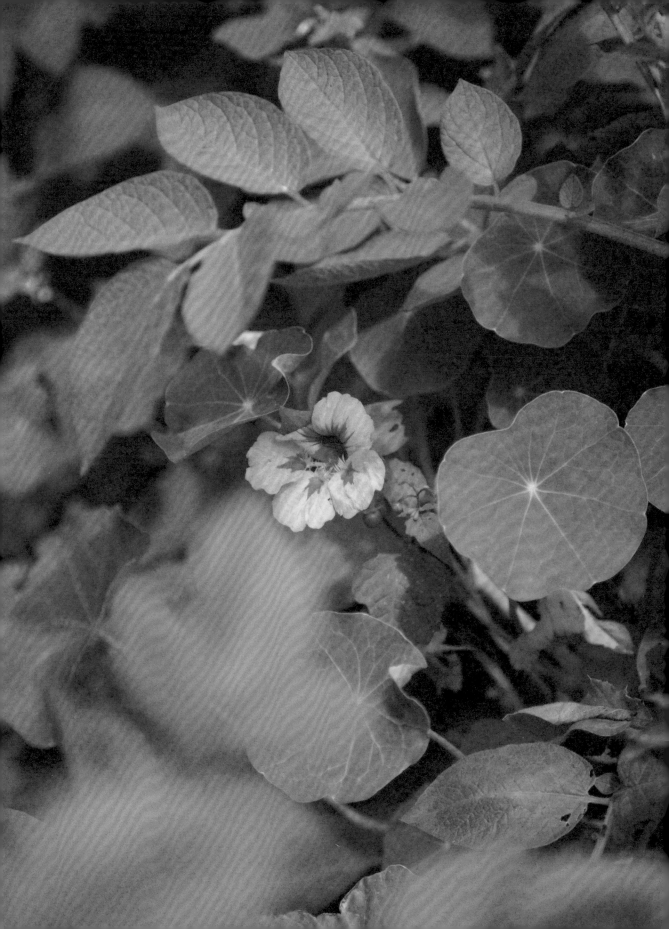

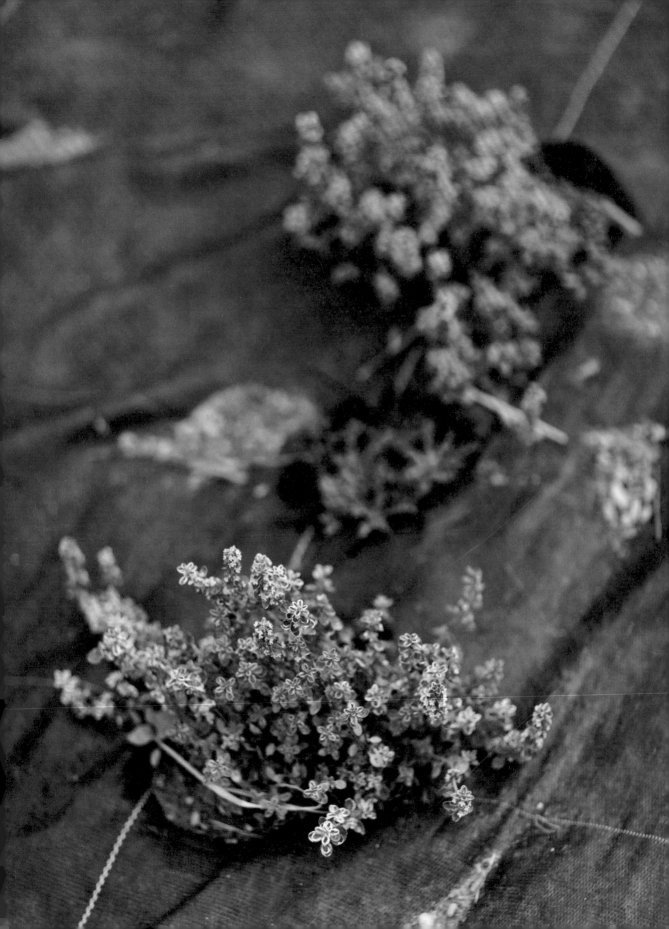

Meanwhile the plants grow thickly to smother most weeds and need only occasional mounding up to prevent the tubers being exposed to the light and turning green.

Large scale (field, smallholding)

Things obviously get easier and easier as your land increases in size. It isn't possible to rear much livestock on a one-acre field, but you can certainly become much more than self-sufficient in vegetables. On this scale you will have to sell your produce, whether fresh or processed.

Indeed, in some particularly fertile areas, such as parts of East Anglia and the West Midlands, an acre of ground is big enough to create a viable market garden – particularly if you put up a polytunnel, which extends the growing season by a few vital weeks at both ends of the growing season.

All the same, you will still need to specialise if you are to make it work. You might not aim to earn loads of money, but a big area will probably require more than the minimal spade, fork and hoe that you need in a garden. Digging is hard work so you will need a rotovator at the very least, while compost and soil improvers such as manure will be needed by the tonne. Water is even heavier, so a quad bike and trailer or small tractor could well be necessary (although it may be possible to arrange for the occasional loan or hire from a bigger neighbour). Once you have got to this stage, however, you open up a new range of possibilities: specialist cereals like oats or spelt (to produce oats or spelt flour) could be viable, particularly if you borrow/rent heavy machinery.

And then there is your labour – anything this size will require a lot of time. This might be a passion and you may think you would do it for fun alone, but the last thing you want is to be slaving away full-time to grow, water and weed your crops, only to find you are effectively losing money. To succeed it needs to be really enjoyable and it will soon lose its gloss when you realise you are subsidising your customers by working for free. Cultivation on this scale still needs careful thought and planning.

With as much ground as this there will be no need to ration space. In fact, the biggest risk is that you plant too much and that it all comes to fruition at once. Not only will you then struggle to sell or at least process the harvest in late summer, but in the run up you will be overwhelmed by the routine maintenance needed to keep your crops watered and free of weeds.

Box schemes are a great way of selling produce as and when it ripens, but they take time to fill and deliver. On the other hand, if you can find hotels, cafés and restaurants that are prepared to take the equivalent of three or four boxes, then the logistics start to tip in your favour. Better still, deal directly with local outlets and grow to order.

GROWING FOR PROFIT?

There are plenty of suppliers, organic and non-organic, who specialise in just one group of vegetables – or even one plant (try Googling 'chilli seeds'). The important thing is to shop around. Seeds are relatively inexpensive, but you can reduce the cost further by ordering with one or more friends. Most packets contain more seeds than one person really needs, and although you can save the spares for the following year, they do slowly lose vitality and it is better to buy fresh supplies each year. If three gardeners germinate one pack of 10 courgette seeds then each will have more than enough for their own family's needs.

As always, farmers' markets can be a great source of inspiration. Local ones will give you a good idea of what grows well in your area, and many stall holders and producers are happy to chat and pass on tips. While on holiday, try to visit other markets for more general ideas about what is popular with customers. For example, what are the best-selling jams or chutneys? Is there a specific unusual flavour combination which works particularly well? (I recently tried a delicious blackcurrant and ginger cordial – a combination that would never have occurred to me.)

In their infinite wisdom, European lawmakers only allow certified plant varieties to be sold. Certification costs several thousand pounds for each strain, which effectively gives control over what we can buy as seed or finished crops to the big seed merchants. It has also greatly restricted the range of ancient plant varieties and threatens some traditional types with extinction.

Fortunately, there are ways of side-stepping the legislation. Both in this country and on the Continent there are charities devoted to saving rare vegetable and fruit varieties. These side-step the certification rules by giving away rare seeds to members or inviting you to take part in growing trials. In Britain the lead organisation is the Henry Doubleday Research Association, which pioneered our organic movement. It has set up the Heritage Seed Library which can supply vegetables which no supermarket could ever stock (www.gardenorganic.org.uk). In France its equivalent, Terre de Semences, was forced out of business by the regulations, but fortunately its place was immediately taken by Association Kokopelli (which has even got the same website – www.terredesemences.com).

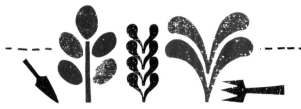

Taking on a bigger and more ambitious approach to growing than simple back-garden production may sound unduly commercial for some people, but it can have hidden advantages. For a start it means you can slowly branch out to produce product ranges and begin to experiment with creating your own brand. This demands lots of creativity, which in itself can be rewarding.

Developing your own products and marketing them will also require you to talk and listen to your customers, pumping all the feedback you acquire into everything you are doing. Once again, the more you can add value to your produce by cooking and refining it, using clever packaging and marketing ideas, the more your margins should increase.

By this stage, however, you will probably need to think about using some sort of commercial premises to carry out this work. It is certainly possible to make 10kg batches of jam or chutney in most domestic kitchens, but try doing this with 100kg or more...

And, of course, at some point around now you will start to need to contact your Council to talk to your local Trading Standards Office for advice on the routine health and hygiene requirements for producing food. Acting on this advice and instituting the various systems and processes required may not be onerous – and you may well be able to rent the use of an existing facility on a part-time basis – but it's something that you do need to investigate.

Know your stuff

Whatever the size of your plot, growing food that you and your family like to eat is key to any success – there's no point growing loads of courgettes if no one likes eating them. Equally, there's no point cultivating crops that can be bought cheaply in the supermarket, but in this case sourcing rare and unusual plant varieties can be particularly worthwhile – a pack of specialist seeds only costs a few pence more than the mainstream equivalents, and after that the plants take no more time and effort to cultivate.

There is still a bewildering range of crops open to the smallholder and it can be difficult to know where to start. There is no way I could cover every option in this book, but here's a quick run through some of the possibilities with some general thoughts on each category.

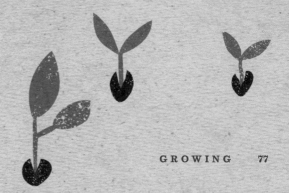

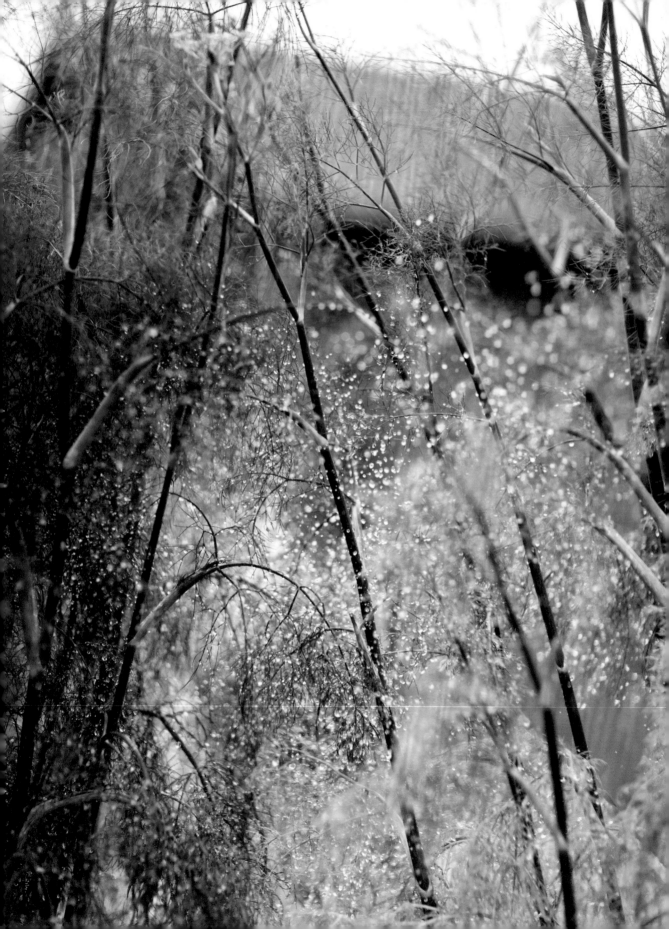

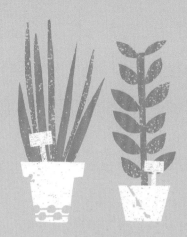
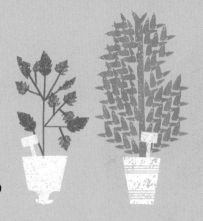

Herbs

Possibly the most useful and most space-saving productive plants you can grow, there are scores of different, tasty herbs to choose from – and usually several varieties of each – so you'll always find some to suit your site and situation.

In many ways herbs are perfect for the small producer. Most are easy to grow and many are very pest-resistant. A little goes a long way, so they also take up very little space. Better still, measured in terms of pence per gram they sell at ridiculously high prices, so even if you only have a few pots standing on a windowsill you can save significant amounts of money on your shopping bill.

More importantly, they pack a great flavour punch, particularly when used fresh. Although we are starting to use more fresh herbs, most people still rely on the jars of dried products which often bear little resemblance to the real McCoy. The difference between a leg of lamb cooked with dried rosemary and one whose flesh has been studded with fresh leaves has to be tasted (and smelled) to be believed.

That said, most herbs also preserve well – it's just that drying isn't always the best solution – so you can save some of your summer bounty for the colder months in a variety of interesting and unusual ways.

Finally, most herbs combine well with other products to create something that is more than the sum of its parts. It doesn't take much imagination to think of ways of mixing them with a variety of meats to make aromatic sausages, roasts or casseroles, flavouring milk to create interesting cheeses or dips or blending with vegetables to make interesting ready meals. Less obvious are ways of locking away their aromas in oil, vinegar, jellies, soaps or cosmetics.

If you do have any intention of selling your produce, it is well worth thinking ahead and finding customers before you start growing. For example, most cuisines rely heavily on half a dozen varieties, so talk to local French or Italian delicatessens and restaurants about whether they would be interested in locally grown organic basil, rosemary, oregano and thyme. Alternatively, Asian outlets may be interested in Thai basil, coriander and fenugreek. They probably already have suppliers, of course, but conventional wholesalers are unlikely to be able to provide some of the more exotic herbs available from the catalogues.

Varieties to grow

In the old days many cottage gardens would boast scores of traditional herbs such as costmary, hyssop, melilot and sweet cicely that are rarely seen today. Most of these largely vanished plants were used for traditional medicines, often dried and steeped in boiling water to produce a weak aromatic tea. You can do the same, of course, but bear in mind that many are an acquired taste. Here are a few of the more common culinary herbs, however:

Basil
This is a relatively delicate-flavoured herb which works particularly well with tomatoes. Although it can't cope with frost, it's easy to grow in pots and it will give a lovely scent to any kitchen windowsill. Almost all the basil sold in this country is the Genovese variety – which is a pity because there are a score of others from around the world. Purple basil will give an interesting dash of colour to a salad, for example, while Greek, Thai and lemon basil all have interesting twists on the basic flavour.

Bay
This comparatively common decorative garden plant (but beware its poisonous look-alike, laurel) is an underused herb in British cooking. The glossy leaves impart a delicate flavour to stocks and bouquet garnis and they are great used in poaching fish. This is a much more substantial plant than most herbs, eventually growing into a fairly large shrub if planted in the right spot – preferably one that is light, airy and south facing. On the other hand, it doesn't cope very well with severe and sharp frosts and so is often grown in containers which are moved indoors or at least into a sheltered spot in harsh weather.

Coriander
A member of the parsley family, this is an essential component in Middle Eastern and Asian cooking. Because of this you can buy it in huge bunches on ethnic market stalls, but nothing beats its flavour when used really fresh – preferably just snipped from the plant and scattered over a dish immediately prior to serving. Again, this is a herb which doesn't dry well, but it is fine frozen or used to flavour oil.

Fennel
This is one of many herbs to have a distinct taste of aniseed and it is traditionally used to flavour fish dishes. Although the flavour is very similar, it should not be confused with Florence fennel which is a different plant, cultivated for its leaf base which swells to make a large bulb that can be eaten raw in salads or cooked as a vegetable.

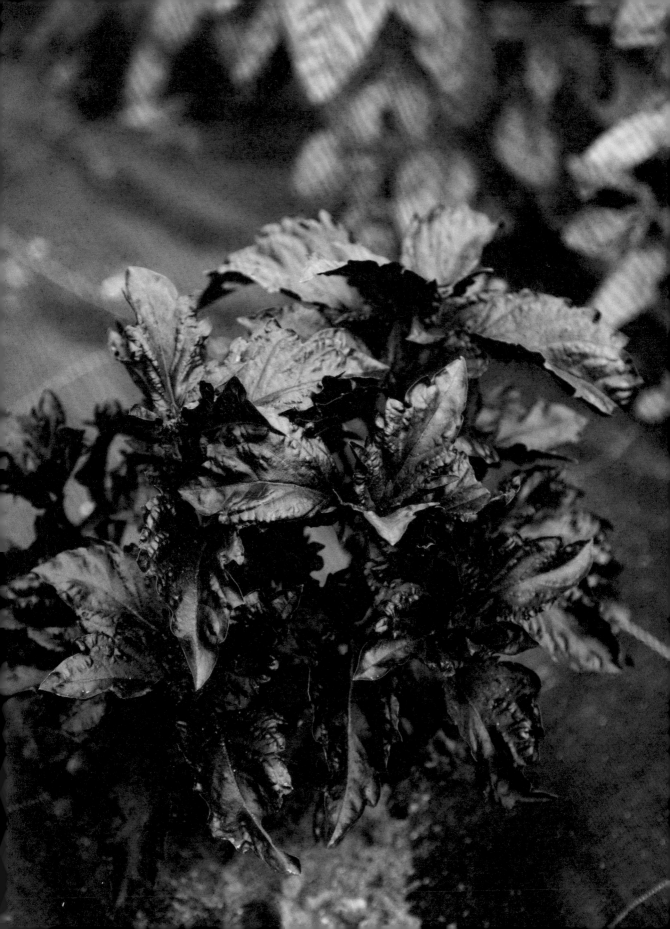

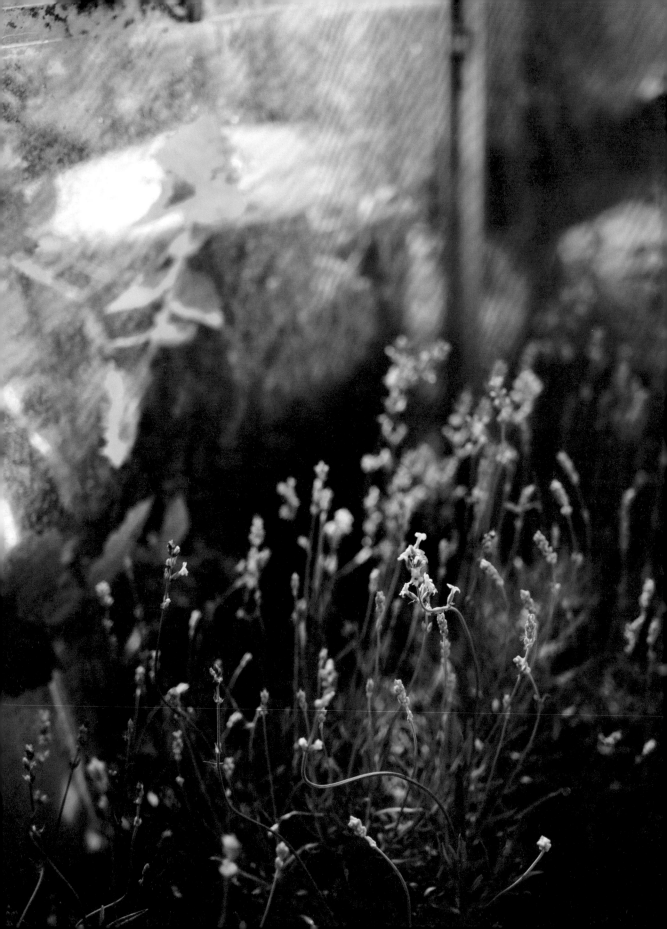

Horseradish

This is another sadly neglected flavouring which oddly works particularly well with robust meats like roast beef and the more delicate flesh of oily fish such as mackerel. This was the traditional source of culinary 'heat' in British cooking until mustard started to become more popular in the eighteenth century. It has declined in popularity a little since, but in Japan the green-fleshed horseradish variety, known as wasabi, is still an essential part of their cuisine.

Horseradish leaves looks somewhat like those of dock and it can be as difficult to eradicate once established. The part to use is the long tap root – but be warned, while grating it gives off astringent juices that can leave you with tears streaming down your cheeks. You may need to wear swimming goggles – and be careful to wash your hands carefully afterwards.

Lavender

Most people think of this as an ornamental, if aromatic, border plant. If they do think of a practical use the most obvious is as an essential oil for cosmetics and toiletries, not to mention pot pourri and pillows, but it is also a fragrant addition to cooking. The leaves and flowers can be used to gently flavour milk puddings, ice cream and biscuits. The traditional French mixed herbs, herbes de Provence à l'ancienne, contains dried lavender, which bumps up the flavour considerably – although experiment judiciously as not everyone likes its perfumed quality.

Lemongrass

Until recently virtually no one in this country had heard of this delicately flavoured stalk, although apparently in the great days of the Empire Queen Victoria was partial to a cup of weak lemongrass tea. It is, of course, an essential ingredient in Thai and Vietnamese cooking, and the increasing popularity of these spicy, aromatic cuisines has brought this herb back into the public attention.

It is both difficult and easy to cultivate: difficult because it needs warmth, easy because, like so many grasses, when it does grow, it grows vigorously. This makes it ideal for a sunny kitchen windowsill. The simplest way to grow your own is to buy a few of the freshest stalks you can find, take them home and put them in a glass of water in the light. Not all will make it, but when little roots appear at the base of the stalk, you can transfer them to a pot of damp compost. New shoots will soon appear.

Marjoram and oregano

There are several types of this herb. The cultivated version, *Origanum majorana*, is generally known as marjoram and is rather more delicate in flavour, but a little better able to cope with the British climate. The wild version, *Origanum vulgare*, is stronger-flavoured, but seems to develop the best flavour in hotter conditions. Easiest of all to to grow is pot marjoram, which is a perennial (keeps growing year after year). Although it usually loses its leaves in winter, it will

DEAD-EASY FOOD DRYING

Although this is one of the oldest ways to store food around the globe, for some reason it never seems to have caught on in Britain. Other nationalities across Europe dry fruit, vegetables, fungi, meat and fish, but we don't – or at least not on any scale. When I think back to my youth, the only dried ingredients I can recall are the tiny green spheres I bought for my pea shooter and dried herbs which were – very significantly – bottled in little jars labelled 'Schwartz' (hardly a British label).

This is surprising, because drying is a very effective way to store food indefinitely. Most food is 70–95 per cent water; this obviously makes it moist and easy to digest, but it does the same for millions of microbes and insects. If you reduce the water content to less than about 20 per cent (preferably lower if keeping is the only consideration), then even bugs find it impossible to consume. In other words, it will keep indefinitely until either reconstituted with water or even chewed as it is (we have enough body fluids in our bodies to rehydrate it internally).

The only reason I can find for this national reluctance to use drying is that it can be mildly tricky in a damp, cool climate. It isn't impossible; after all, until 30 years ago we relied on exactly the same principles to dry our laundry (I still do, at least in summer). More importantly, every summer farmers cut and bale millions of tonnes of hay using solar energy as the main preserving agent.

The basic principles are very simple. Temperature is less important than the flow of dry (or dry-ish) air around the subject matter. So as anyone who regularly hangs out washing will tell you, clothes dry quickest on a windy rather than a hot still day. Also, one of the best ways to slow the process down is if the drying material overlaps. If slices of vegetable, meat or fungi are piled on top of each other, moulds will soon start to develop between the touching surfaces. So just as laundry dries faster when stretched taut on the line, so food will dessicate best when every surface is surrounded by an air-flow. This is also why farmers toss their hay several times to ensure all-round dryness before baling.

With these principles in mind, drying food is fairly easy. As with hay, the biggest challenge is the race to beat the fungi and bacteria which are also determined to consume your precious produce before it becomes too dry to support life. This can be tricky in our mercurial climate, but it's not impossible. There are two broad methods – to use the natural elements or to employ artificial heat.

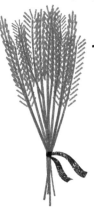

✔ USING NATURE – THE SUN AND WIND

Most cultures which use drying on a big scale rely on the elements. This is obviously easy in Mediterranean or African nations. It's tricky, but still possible here. After all, our farmers manage to do it year after year in even the wettest summers by keeping a careful eye on the weather forecast for a 'window' of a few days.

If you have a clear hot spell at the end of summer, you can usually get away with putting your thinly sliced produce on wire racks in the full glare of the sun, but this often isn't enough. A better solution is to build a simple solar drying cabinet by painting a wooden box black inside, tilting it at about a 30-degree angle towards the south west and covering it with a sheet of glass, ensuring there is plenty of ventilation at both the top and bottom of the chamber. The glass and black colouring will raise the internal temperature 20 or 30 degrees above those outside and natural convection currents will move a steady stream of warm air across the produce.

Alternatively, less rot-prone materials, such as bunches of oregano or lavender, can simply be hung from the roof in a room or dry outbuilding out of direct sunlight. This can even work for strips of meat if you aim to make South African 'biltong' or Native American 'pemmican' (the latter is a mix of dried lean meat and berries with added fat). Meat is quick to taint, however (and obviously needs to be kept free of flies), so it is usually better to do this indoors in the dry of a heated home.

✔ SCIENTIFIC SOLUTIONS

If you can't rely on the elements, artificial heat could be the answer. The problem here is to avoid overheating. Remember, the most effective drier is air-flow, not high temperature, which can often degrade the material (think of freeze-dried coffee which relies on extremely dry cold air to preserve the essential oils and flavours). Some people suggest putting produce in the lowest possible oven setting and leaving the door open, but in my experience this is usually too much.

You can buy fairly cheap desiccating machines online, but these also are often set too high and toast their contents. It is often just as easy (and much cheaper) to concoct your own system. I use fine welded mesh (you can buy small sheets from builders' merchants) and snip the corners to make a crude tray. Then cover these with thin strips of produce and stack them on top of a wood-burning stove. Alternatively, you could put them in an airing cupboard – or even use a low-wattage light bulb mounted in a biscuit tin as a mild heat source to get the air flowing.

As your produce dries, keep a close eye on it, rotating it regularly to ensure it dries evenly and that nothing over-cooks. When conditions are right the whole process can be amazingly quick – only a few hours' duration in some cases – and, depending on the product, the end result should keep for up to several years if stored in an airtight container.

spring up again in the same spot in much the same way as mint. It's great scattered fresh on roasts or even in salads (golden marjoram has a milder flavour, which makes it ideal for this). Marjoram and oregano also freeze well and are good for flavouring oils, but unlike most herbs the coarser, more powerful varieties are arguably improved by drying.

Mint

The British always associate this vigorous herb with lamb and summer drinks like Pimm's and mint julep, but it has plenty of other uses, too. The Arabs drink copious amounts of sweet mint tea made by infusing the fresh herb in hot water, and they also scatter it over all manner of hot and cold dishes. It dries moderately well, freezes better and, of course, makes a great savoury jelly to serve with hot or cold meats. It is very easy to grow – in fact too easy. Although it apparently dies every winter, new shoots spring up the next spring and once established the biggest problem is stopping it taking over. Some people get round the problem by growing it in pots, others plant it in an old bucket with the bottom knocked out and bury it in the ground to act as a barrier to prevent the roots spreading.

Parsley

Until recently parsley was probably the most heavily used herb in classic British cooking. It works particularly well with fish and dairy (for example, cod in parsley sauce), but it is also notable for reducing the smell of garlic. There are several types, but the two commonest are curly (until recently this was the most popular in Britain, perhaps because it is more decorative) and plain – or 'French' – which chefs generally believe has more flavour.

Rosemary

We think of this woody perennial as a Mediterranean herb, but it will survive outdoors in a pot or border for years in British winters. It is rich in essential oils and it gives a powerful flavour punch to many dishes, but particularly red meats. It is traditionally associated with lamb, but it works brilliantly with beef and venison too. Or try coating a mixture of winter root vegetables in olive oil, scattering with plenty of rosemary, black pepper and salt and roasting in a hot oven. To my mind it doesn't dry well and is best used fresh, but fortunately as an evergreen its thick waxy leaves are available for picking all year round. That said, rosemary is also great for flavouring oils, vinegars and (a particular and unusual favourite) jellies (see the recipe on p.228).

Sage

As a pig fanatic, this is obviously one of my favourite herbs because it has long been used as the backbone of many great pork dishes. Combined with onion it also makes the classic poultry stuffing, but it's got far more uses than this. Try baking a marrow, scooping out the insides and blending them with a mixture of breadcrumbs, chopped onion and sage, then returning to the oven with a dusting

HITTING THE HERB MARKET

Although fresh herbs – particularly growing in pots – now regularly appear in shops, there is plenty of scope to harness their flavours in a range of ways, many of which are vastly superior to the traditional dried varieties on which British cooks tend to rely. Certainly the flavours of one or two herbs, such as marjoram and oregano, seem to be every bit as good when dried, but this is because they are lower in volatile oils so the process concentrates the original flavour rather than degrades it. The problem with many of the aromatic herbs, such as basil, is that the essential oils that give them their appeal are largely lost in the drying process.

The answer for these herbs is to trap the aromas by locking them in liquids. Many are particularly good infused in oils or vinegars, for example basil oil and tarragon vinegar. These are reasonably well known, but similar effects can be achieved using jellies, chutneys and pickles. Apple jelly is an ideal base because on its own it is relatively bland, but it readily assumes the flavour of rosemary. A delicate herb chutney can make an unusual accompaniment for oily fish, while a mixed pickle is an interesting relish for hot or cold meats.

Another solution is to adapt the Italian recipe for pesto. Instead of grinding basil, pine nuts, Parmesan and garlic with sea salt and olive oil, try substituting parsley, hazelnuts and Cheddar for the first three ingredients.

Of course it goes without saying that for me mixing herbs with pork to make unusual sausages is the perfect way of adding value to both. Even something as simple as putting a big bunch of fresh herbs in with a Christmas turkey is a great marketing tip. As your customer opens the packaging they are greeted with a huge waft of delicious aromas. Or you can go one step further and prepare oven-ready dishes, coating roasting joints or fresh root vegetables with freshly chopped herbs, possibly mixed with honey and fruit juices to ensure they stick fairly evenly.

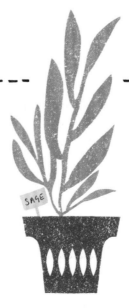

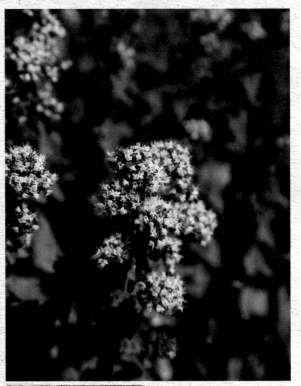

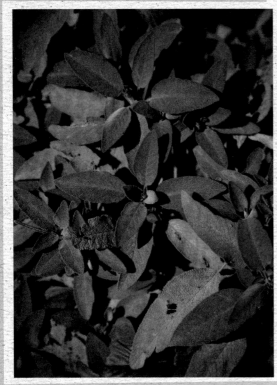

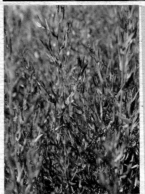

MOST HERBS, such as SAGE, OREGANO and TARRAGON, are PERFECT for the small producer. HERBS are EASY to GROW and... a LITTLE goes a LONG WAY, so they also take up VERY LITTLE space.

of more breadcrumbs over the top. It does have an extremely powerful flavour, however, so use it judiciously. The benefit of this is that a small bush or even a pot will supply all the leaves that you are likely to need for your own use – although its furry silvery green and purple foliage make it such an attractive plant you may well want to use it to brighten up your borders.

Sorrel

Whether you count this as a herb or a salad vegetable is debatable. Its distinct lemony flavour is still sufficiently subtle for it to be used in much larger quantities than most herbs – although more moderately than, for example, spinach. It is popular in French kitchens, where it frequently appears in soups and omelettes, but it also works well raw in salads, particularly when cut young.

Tarragon

Another classic French herb which is much less popular here, for some reason. This is a classic herb to serve with chicken (try mixing it with cream cheese and sliding this paste between the skin and flesh of a chicken before roasting). It has a delicate flavour which also works well with fish (stuff the body cavity of a trout or bass with the leaves before baking or poaching), although it also works well in omelettes and mixed with butter as an accompaniment to steak. This is another herb with two distinct varieties. The most vigorous is 'Russian', but 'French' is the one to grow because its taste is streets

ahead. It is a perennial herb which comes up again and again in the same spot, but it may need a little protection in a hard winter – perhaps a covering of straw or fleece. It doesn't dry particularly well, but it is brilliant when steeped in vinegar to produce a delicately scented condiment which also works well in salad dressings.

Thyme

This is another perennial that dies back in winter, but which usually retains enough leaves to use fresh around the year, so although it dries moderately well there is no real need to do so. Like other oily herbs, it has a robust flavour, so you don't need huge amounts in any dish and it roasts well with both meat and vegetables – particularly when combined with the acidity of lemon. It is also the famous partner for parsley in stuffings.

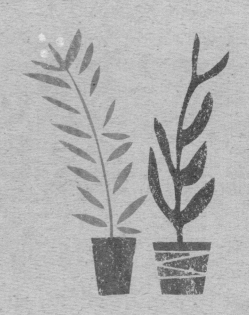

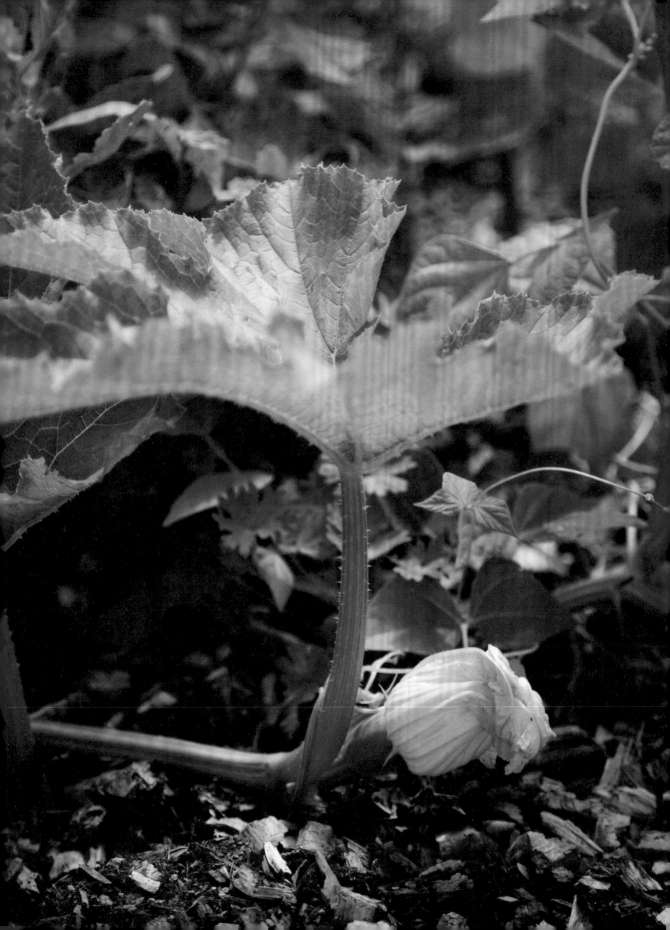

Grow outside the box

It is incredibly satisfying to grow anything, even if it is only carrots, beans or potatoes, but, that said, it is even more rewarding when you cultivate an old favourite that's just a little bit different.

One of the best ways you can do this is to seek out less commonly grown seed varieties to improve on the range of produce available on shop shelves. Here I am talking about producing something for your own purposes which is superior to the ones you would normally encounter.

There are very good reasons most retailers stock a relatively limited range of each type of vegetable. If you are a big supermarket, qualities like high productivity, long shelf-life, uniformity and appealing looks are critical.

This means that while some traditional varieties might not fit the top priorities of the big retailers, rarer seed strains might have qualities which are better suited to your needs. Most obviously they might not be high yielding, but make up for this with taste and texture. Others may be disease- or pest-resistant (which is important if you want to grow without chemicals), while growing a range of varieties can extend your growing season or make the most of limited space (for example by growing tumbling cherry tomatoes in a hanging basket or climbing cucumbers up a trellis).

Beetroot
Instead of growing spherical, deep red beetroot, how about cultivating the sweet-fleshed and striking 'Chiogga', which has concentric rings of red and white? Or 'Cylindra', which produces longer, thinner, roots, which makes them ideal for lighter soils. The list of possibilities is almost endless, so the best advice is to spend time researching catalogues, preferably from some of the specialist seed importers rather than the three or four biggest British firms.

Broad beans
Unlike most beans, these are very hardy, even tolerating a bit of frost, so they are thus one of the first crops of the year.

They tend to be looked down on as a bit coarse and unpalatable, but this is because commercial growers sell by weight, so they tend to pick them when they are really a bit too big. Then, not only do you need to pod them, but sometimes also need to peel the beans themselves. This is such a pity because when picked young and tender they are as sweet and tender as a pea.

Broccoli
This is another vegetable with far more varieties than most people realise – probably because most never appear in the shops. The vegetable which very loosely resembles a green cauliflower is technically calabrese, not broccoli, but they are closely related and need broadly the same cultivation techniques. True broccoli appears most often as purple sprouting broccoli and to my mind has a better flavour and texture – when cooked well (it is easy to overdo this). One of the great attractions of this group is that they are very hardy and will provide plenty of green vegetables through the colder months. It freezes well after blanching, but is at its best fresh when it is most needed in the depths of winter.

Cabbage
For many centuries the cabbage was one of the mainstays of the British diet – and with good reason. It has a very long growing season and if you grow a range of varieties you can harvest it virtually year round. Unfortunately, for many people the cabbage has been ruined as a vegetable by being boiled until it is little more than a grey pulp. This is a tragedy, because there is a fantastic range of colours, tastes and textures available, although usually no more than three or four feature on supermarket shelves. It also pickles well (think of German sauerkraut or the fiery Korean kimchi).

Carrot
This is such a staple that we take it for granted. The name of the variety rarely features and in the shops they come in just the one standard shape and colour – the only real difference is generally whether they are sold young in bunches with the leaves still on or a little older, topped and tailed. This is such a pity because there is a huge range of shapes and colours. Better still, with a little imagination and research you can grow and harvest them around the year, making carrots an ideal element for box schemes. Finally, they are far more versatile than most people realise. We tend to eat them raw or steamed, but they also make a good pickling ingredient and some excellent chutneys.

Courgette
These are very simple to grow and can be extremely prolific – so much so that you almost always end up with an embarrassment of marrows when you can't keep up with their output. For some reason almost the only ones you see in shops are a uniform dark green, gherkin-shaped. This is a great pity because there are hundreds of varieties of all shapes

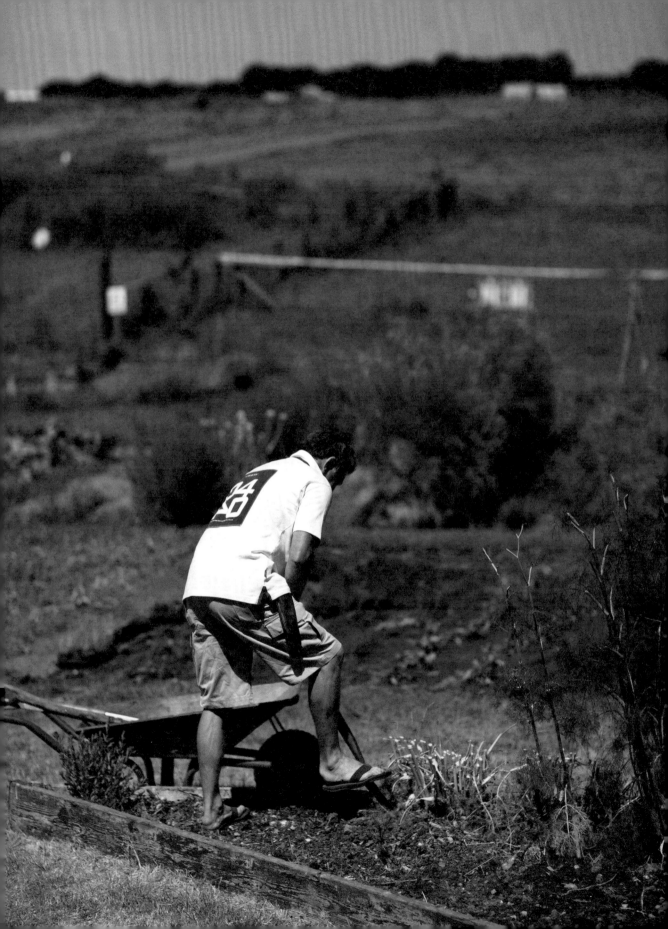

and sizes. For example, why not grow gold versions to give colour to the dinner table? Alternatively there are wonderful globe versions such as 'Tondo di Nizza', which you harvest when the size of a tennis ball, which are perfect for stuffing. Or there is the ribbed variety, 'Costata Romanesco', which many chefs consider to have the best flavour of all. Also, don't overlook the flowers, which are so short-lived they never appear in shops yet are a real delicacy when stuffed, dipped in batter and deep fried.

French bean
These are more delicate than broad or runner beans. There are hundreds of varieties and they come in all sizes, shapes and colours. The most familiar to most people is a small stringless type, the Kenyan, which is eaten whole. These do grow here, but most of those eaten here are flown in from abroad. As a result they are relatively expensive, so growing your own saves thousands of road and air miles over the shop variety.

Bigger types can also be grown for their seeds, however, which can be dried to produce haricot beans for the winter. Like most beans and peas these plants can be incredibly productive in a small space, so you can even coax enough for a few meals from a couple of plants in a pot on a windowsill. Their biggest problem is that they are very delicate and the slightest hint of frost will kill them. Indeed, if they are planted too early they will also struggle and they tend to fall victim to slugs, snails and voles.

Garlic
It seems incredible that only 50 years ago the great cookery writer Elizabeth David was urging us not to be scared of this vegetable and was suggesting we perk up a salad by rubbing a peeled clove around the inside of the bowl. Thanks to the revolution in British cooking over the last half century, during which we have cheerfully borrowed from every cuisine under the sun, the idea of living without garlic is unthinkable. It grows well here, too, and the taste of creamy fresh garlic straight from the garden is much milder than the older versions you find in the shops. As well as being an essential culinary ingredient, it stores well if the leaves are plaited together, but you can also process it in a huge range of interesting ways – such as pickling or smoking.

Kale
This is another great hardy vegetable which provides plenty of green foliage through the colder months when many other crops are long gone. Older varieties tended to be a little bitter, which may explain why it has struggled to achieve popularity. Newer strains are much sweeter, however, and thanks to television chefs promoting Italian varieties like cavalo nero, kale has at last started to become more fashionable.

Leek
This has indelible associations with Wales, but it grows well almost anywhere in Britain. Indeed, it is easiest of the

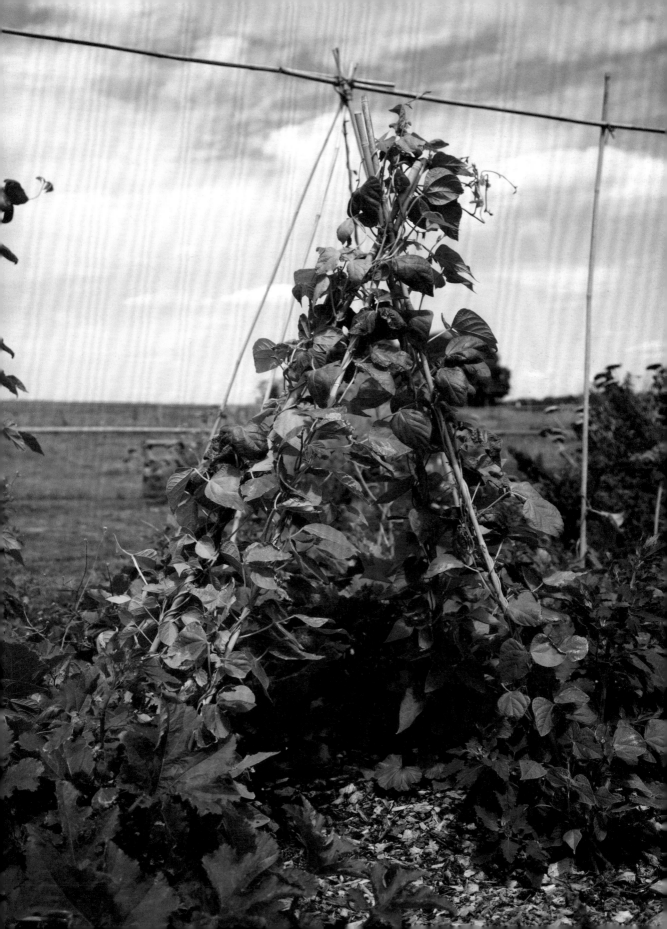

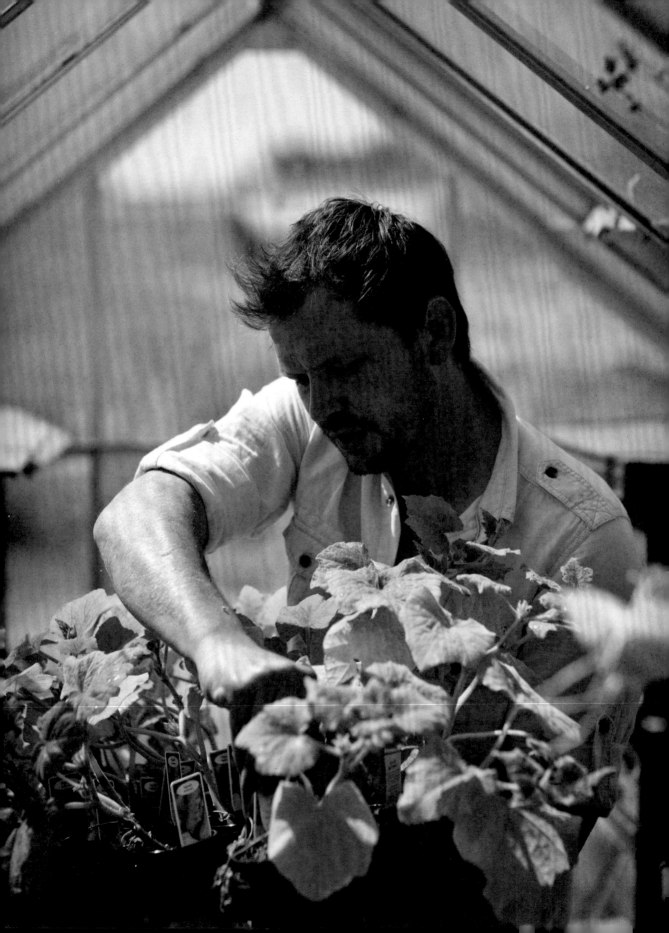

onion family to cultivate and is particularly valuable because it is very hardy and will happily sit in the ground well into the New Year. Indeed, if you stagger your plantings it has a six-month harvesting season. It might not be quite as important as garlic or onions as a culinary 'base' ingredient, but it is delicious in its own right (try it steamed and served with toasted sesame seed oil).

Onion

Although these are a completely vital ingredient in almost every cuisine you can think of, it is questionable whether they are worth growing – particularly if space is short. They are so readily available and cheap in the shops that I can't help thinking the space and effort would be better taken up with something else. On the other hand, they are such an essential ingredient and so easy to grow from sets (miniature onions raised from seed) that it seems a pity to leave them out of any kitchen garden. One compromise might be to find an unusual variety – or possibly to cultivate the closely related shallot which arguably has a better flavour and is – inexplicably – much more expensive.

Parsnip

This is a gorgeous hardy root vegetable which, far from being damaged by frost, is supposed to be actually improved by chilling. It is naturally high in sugars, which means that when roast or fried it becomes positively sweet. Indeed, during World War II it was mixed with flavourings to produce an – admittedly unconvincing – mock banana. Its main drawback is that it is fairly slow growing and if you want big roots you need to give each root a fair amount of space. In other words, it can take up a lot of bed for a long time.

Pea

Like beans, peas are relatively high in protein and in the past were grown principally for drying to store summer energy for the winter. Today, of course, we think of them almost entirely as a fresh crop, helped, no doubt, by the fact that they store so well in a freezer – and this is one area where commercial farmers have definitely got the product right. They grow particularly small, sweet varieties which are then harvested, processed and frozen within a few hours. This makes growing conventional peas for sale a bit of a headache because most consumers are so used to the cheapness and convenience of the frozen product that it is difficult to persuade them to go back to traditional shelling – and even more difficult to get the peas to them as quickly as they ought to move from plant to pan. That said, there is nothing like a really fresh pea pulled straight from the pod, so these are brilliant for personal use.

One answer is to turn to those varieties which are designed to be eaten pod and all. Mangetout are eaten whole – as are sugar snap peas. These are all early cropping (the former are often known as snow peas), easy to cultivate and heavy cropping – which is why I've never understood why they are sold in such small, expensive packets.

CASE STUDY ≫

CASE STUDY GARLIC

Glen Allingham comes from GENERATIONS of FARMERS. His father Was Born on a MIXED BEDFORDSHiRe farm.

While stationed in Scotland during National Service with the RAF, Glen's father fell in love with the local baker's daughter. After relocating there, together they bought Craiggie Farm in 1962, a couple of years after Glen was born, and slowly they began to specialise first in pigs and later in seed potatoes.

Glen's wife, Gilli, joined the family at the Scottish farm by pure chance. 'I used to cook for people on shooting and fishing holidays,' she says. 'I worked for Glen's uncle and aunt and through this was invited to cater at a family wedding in Norfolk, where I met Glen – the family joke is that he "married below stairs",' she laughs.

From the mid-90s, though, Glen became aware that the 200-acre farm was too small for financial comfort. 'We had had a couple of bad potato years, so it was clear we had to do something more profitable if our daughters were ever to take over the farm – that is, if they want to,' explained Gilli. The obvious solution was to buy more land, but because they were effectively landlocked by large estates on all sides there was little prospect of success there. As a result, by the time the couple took over the farm in 1998, Glen was actively seeking to diversify into an area of production where acreage was less of an issue.

The breakthrough came at a meeting organised by the Scottish Agricultural College in Inverness. The college was looking for farmers to run trials of unusual crops including daffodils, borage and garlic. On the spur of the moment, Glen put his hand up and returned home to announce to Gilli that they were going to be growing garlic the following season.

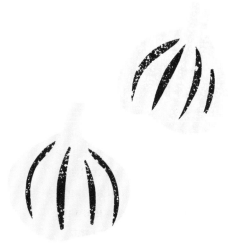

In the first year the college sourced the seed for the couple, finding three hard-necked varieties they thought might withstand the rigours of a Scottish growing season. One was from the Isle of Wight, another from Austria and the final one revelled in the name 'Russian Red'.

The couple were lucky in that as a trial the college paid for their labour and the rental on a patch of their land, but it was still backbreaking work. 'We had to hand-plant, hand-weed and hand-lift the whole lot,' recalls Gilli.

Fortunately it grew well and in the end they bought the crop straight back and sold most of it at their local farmers' market. They kept back some cloves to plant the following year, but lost most of them to a botrytis infection. However, by now the couple had the bit between their teeth and they began to look for varieties better suited to the Scottish climate.

'We came across some people in Canada who were growing a hard-necked variety called 'Music',' says Gilli. 'We figured that although their weather conditions were more extreme than ours – there's snow on the ground until April and summers are much hotter – conditions were not that dissimilar and we ordered enough to plant five acres.'

In 2000 Glen and Gilli started the Really Garlicky Company, and for the first ten years all profits have been ploughed into the business. Although the amount of land dedicated to garlic has grown steadily over the years, it still represents only a small portion of the farm. This is partly because garlic is susceptible to various fungal diseases, so it has to be rotated every year and the ground cannot be replanted for five years. As a result, in 2010 the home farm had 35 acres of garlic, 150 acres of barley and 70 acres of wheat, while there were 150 acres of potatoes on local rented land.

As with all crops there are good and bad years, but even in a great season the problems don't end with the harvest. The lifted garlic bulbs are very moist and need curing before being sold, in the same way that onions are dried. Another problem is that hard-necked varieties don't store as well as the French soft-necked strains, so the Allinghams only sell fresh garlic from July to December. Despite this, upmarket supermarkets buy as many bulbs as the couple can supply and are happy to pay a premium for a British-grown crop.

Of course, not every bulb is perfect, but the Allinghams have found a way to turn waste into profit. 'All reject bulbs are puréed then turned into a growing list of value-added products such as aioli, garlic bread, garlic cream cheese, garlic oatcakes, sweet chilli and garlic mayonnaise and salad dressings. 'Garlic butter is our biggest line,' beams Gilli.

There are some downsides to success; the level of paperwork is huge. Obviously the factory has to pass routine hygiene inspections, but increasingly traceability is important, too. Yet Gilli still loves the unexpected turn Glen took back in 1998. 'I trained as a cook and married a farmer – what could be better than him growing the raw ingredients for me to turn into a range of delicious products?'

Potatoes

Ever since the seventeenth century potatoes have played a vital role in first the British and later the world's diet. However, even the most expensive organic varieties are so comparatively cheap to buy in supermarkets that it is questionable whether they are worth growing at home – particularly if space is limited. That said, they are very easy to cultivate and on a larger scale they can be a good way of breaking up compacted soil and helping to choke weeds. If you do decide to grow these, it is important to choose a variety you like. Unless you have a really big garden, I would avoid maincrops (they take up too much space for too long) – best leave them to farmers with big fields and heavy machinery.

New and salad potatoes are different, though. The first are so delicious when really fresh that I think they can rank along with strawberries as a seasonal delicacy. Also, they will be ready for lifting in June or July, leaving space for frost-sensitive crops like beans. The second are also expensive (for potatoes) and again, when cooked within a few minutes of lifting from the soil they are delicious and to my mind one of the great joys of summer. Although you need space to get a good crop, you can get two or three meals-worth from a big bin or plastic bag filled with compost on a balcony. One unusual, but satisfying, idea is to pick a sheltered spot and plant one of these with a salad variety in late summer (you can use sprouting potatoes from the supermarket if you can't find genuine seed). Protect from frost and harvest on Christmas morning to give the meal a little extra flavour and significance.

Pumpkins

The British have never really taken to the squash family, which is a puzzle because they are a great staple across much of the rest of the world. African and Caribbean cuisine, for example, rely heavily on various members of this huge family and, after all, pumpkins are America's unofficial national vegetable. Over here, however, their supply is limited largely to a brief annual appearance of big, bright orange 'Halloween' fruits in October.

I have a feeling this sad state of affairs may soon change. The wonderful butternut is beginning to appear more widely in shops and supermarkets and you sometimes see other types in ethnic stores. There is certainly a huge range of possible shapes, sizes, colours and flavours to turn to and they are easy to grow and prolific. Many – such as patty pans – are quick to mature and great in stir-fries, while others dry well to make unusual decorations.

Radishes

In this country we tend to use radishes only as a salad vegetable, but they are actually much more versatile than that.

We are used to the small red and white roots, but there are oriental varieties which can be black, white- or red-fleshed. These can also be much larger – 'Mooli', for example, can easily reach 30cm in length and work well in stir fries. Others,

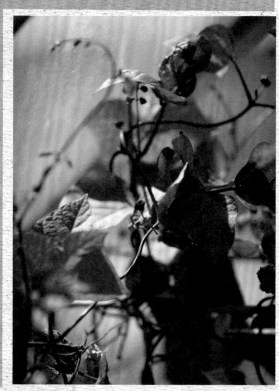

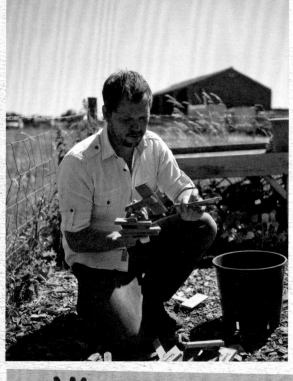

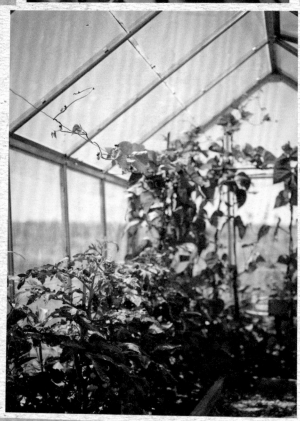

growing a range of VARIETIES CAN EXTEND your growing SEASON or MAKE the MOST of LIMITED space.

such as winter radish, will grow and crop during the colder months when most other plants are dormant. They are also extremely fast-growing, maturing in as little as four weeks, although the bigger and larger types will take twice as long.

Runner beans

It is said that this is the most productive crop you can have, and for that reason these are a real favourite of home-growers and allotment holders. Just one wigwam of five or six poles will quickly be covered with climbing beans that will produce a prodigious number of pods throughout the summer – more than most families could consume.

A pretty wigwam of canes or willow is ornamental too, particularly when festooned with red or white flowers, so these can look lovely dotted around the beds in your back garden.

Spinach

A great garden staple and one of the most versatile of green vegetables, it makes a great vegetable and salad crop. Annual spinach cut young works well in salads, but it also cooks brilliantly when it becomes a little more mature.

The other type that is available is perpetual spinach, which actually belongs to a different family, being related to chard and beetroot. Like those vegetables, it has a thick midrib on the leaves and a slightly coarser flavour, so it is generally cooked for best results, although the baby leaves can be eaten in salads.

Swiss chard

This is a vegetable that is starting to be widely cultivated but is still a comparative rarity in shops because it doesn't travel well and is best eaten freshly picked.

It is a hardy plant that can produce welcome greens throughout the winter. The flavour is like coarse spinach, but it also has a thick stalk, so it's usually best to cook this separately from the leaves (steam these and serve with plenty of melted butter and black pepper – delicious!). Chard can also be very ornamental, so it's great in a small garden where you want dual-purpose vegetables, especially varieties such as 'Bright Lights' which has a range of almost garishly coloured red, yellow and white stalks.

Tomatoes

These are so important in our daily diets that they are one of the first things many beginner veg gardeners start with, but again it is questionable whether it is worth growing this warm-weather crop. They are certainly not difficult, but they are cheap to buy in the shops and they often struggle to ripen in our climate.

If you want fruit through the summer, indoor tomatoes will virtually always produce a heavier yield, earlier, than the outdoor varieties. Generally, however, you will almost always get a glut of fruit at the end of summer, but then this can easily be turned into a range of delicious products, from passata to green tomato chutney or even used in prepared dishes.

This is certainly a case where it is worth poring over the catalogues to find something which suits your needs. You will find a vast range of sizes, from beefsteak to plum to cherry. Almost all shop tomatoes are red spheres of one size or another, but if you check the catalogues there is a bewildering variety of shapes and colours (the Italian word '*pomodoro*' actually means golden apple). If you only have a small patio or even a hanging basket, try a tumbling yellow cherry variety, for example, while beefsteak varieties such as 'Marmande' will do well in a growbag on a balcony or roof.

Turnip

It seems strange to think that until the eighteenth century this was the root vegetable that formed the mainstay of the British diet. It is now sadly neglected, mainly because when it does appear in shops it tends to be as a large, rather woody root. In fact it has real potential in the garden because it is quick growing, taking only eight weeks to produce golfball-sized sweet roots which are delicious cooked whole alongside a Sunday roast. In the interim, the leaves from the thinnings make an interesting salad leaf. The downside is that, unlike the bigger versions, the little roots have a high water content which means they wilt and shrivel quickly once harvested. This is obviously no problem if it's for your personal consumption, but it can be a real problem if you are trying to sell them in a shop or even a market stall.

FIRST FIND YOUR MARKET...

Whatever scale you are working to, it is important to work out where your delicate seedlings are going to go. Timing is obviously important – there is no point proudly putting out young French beans for sale at Easter or in August. They need to be about 15cm tall at about the time of the last frost (ask locally and check meteorological records on the internet).

Also, do some gentle market research. Talk to keen local gardeners and the Women's Institute about what grows best locally, what they might be interested in and what they find difficult to locate. You should also speak (gently and tactfully) to garden centres about best-selling lines (flowers or vegetables?) and the typical profile of their customers. Better still, start off by making direct offers to friends and acquaintances to raise a few seedlings of their choice.

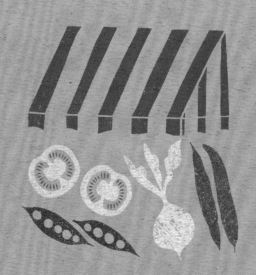

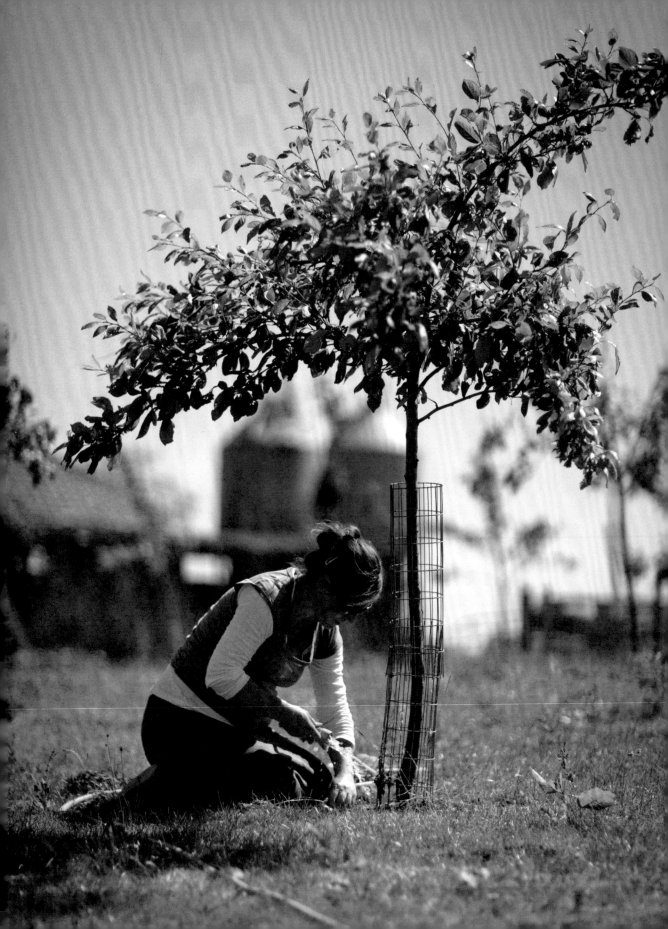

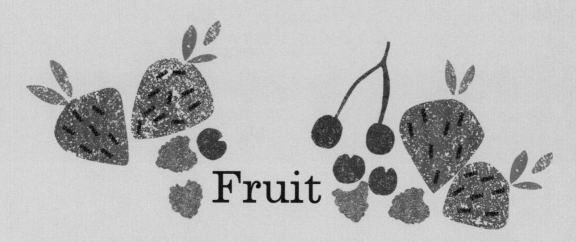

Fruit

There's nothing lovelier than plucking an apple from a tree in autumn or gathering succulent strawberries from your very own plants, but growing fruit can be a lot more demanding and problematic than you might think.

To be able to harvest enough fruit to see you through the summer or to sell or give away outside of your own family, you do need a lot of plants – and of course fruit trees and bushes can be pretty big, which rules out planting many types in small gardens. Even in bigger plots you could get a steady stream of vegetables and a bigger harvest year round from a raised bed covering the same area.

If you're growing organically, this brings with it another set of issues. Without chemical sprays, you will produce a great deal of misshapen and blemished apples and pears. These may be perfectly edible, but they will be very difficult to sell. Also, the most popular varieties of hard fruit – such as Granny Smith, Golden Delicious and Gala – don't grow well here. (Although this is not so for the Bramley, which is almost the only cooking apple you can buy in most shops.) It is a

shame because Britain was once a great apple- and pear-growing nation. We had hundreds of native varieties and much of Kent, Herefordshire and Gloucestershire was covered with orchards.

On the other hand, a lot of established gardens, particularly in the countryside, come with a few apple and pear trees – some even with a small orchard. There are also times when it is definitely worth planting new trees. For example, in the past plums were often planted in hedges on the grounds that this is effectively no-man's-land. This works particularly well with some of the older, thorny plum varieties, which make a dense, fairly impenetrable windbreak while also yielding copious amounts of fruit. Alternatively, if you live in a traditional apple- or pear-growing region, you might feel sufficiently motivated to want to try to save a traditional regional variety.

Another possibility is to make use of a south-facing wall to grow an unusual or delicate fruit tree. This works particularly well if you train it along wires to make an espalier or fan. If you are fortunate enough to have a suitable wall, it seems a waste to plant familiar fruit trees when you could be growing something a little more exotic such as apricots, peaches, cherries or eating grapes.

If you do have trees there is plenty you can do with the glut of fruit that will arrive every autumn. Both apples and pears can be pulped and pressed with inexpensive equipment to make delicious fresh juice. If you pop this in jars with airlocks and leave it for a couple of months you will get wonderful scrumpy and perry (the best comes from special varieties which are too tart and high in tannin to eat or cook with, but which impart a superior flavour after fermentation).

Apricot (and peach)

Although really a warm-weather tree, several varieties of hardier apricots have been developed which are capable of cropping well in Britain – although ideally they need a south-facing wall and frost-protection in winter. Peaches are even more delicate, but there are a few hardier strains which will not only survive but will also fruit heavily here. Covering the tree with a polythene or fleece sheet in late autumn helps, and this should only be removed when the buds unfurl and risk of frost has passed. The fruit is delicious eaten straight from the plant, but it also makes great jams and chutneys.

Blueberry

Until recently this American berry was virtually unknown here, then someone discovered its antioxidants, flavinoids and high vitamin C content, it became a 'wonder food' and sales rocketed. It needs an ericaceous soil, so unless you have an acidic soil it is best grown in pots of appropriate compost. This makes it ideal for patios and balconies. Check your variety carefully if you only have room for one plant, though, as it needs to be a self-fertile one or you won't get any fruit.

Blackberry

At first glance the idea of planting blackberries when these are so widely available for free along towpaths, country lanes and footpaths seems ludicrous, but in actual fact the cultivated versions are bigger and generally sweeter than the wild fruit.

A much better use, however, is to incorporate them in hedges around your property, improving its impenetrability to humans, livestock and the wind, while also producing copious soft fruit for humans and wildlife alike in the autumn.

Cranberry

This is an acid- and damp-loving berry. In its native America it is grown commercially in huge boggy fields, but as a straggling trailing plant it also grows well in hanging baskets, which is, of course, ideal for many space-starved gardens and flats. Better still, as well as the dark red berries in autumn, in mid-summer it is festooned with pretty pink flowers.

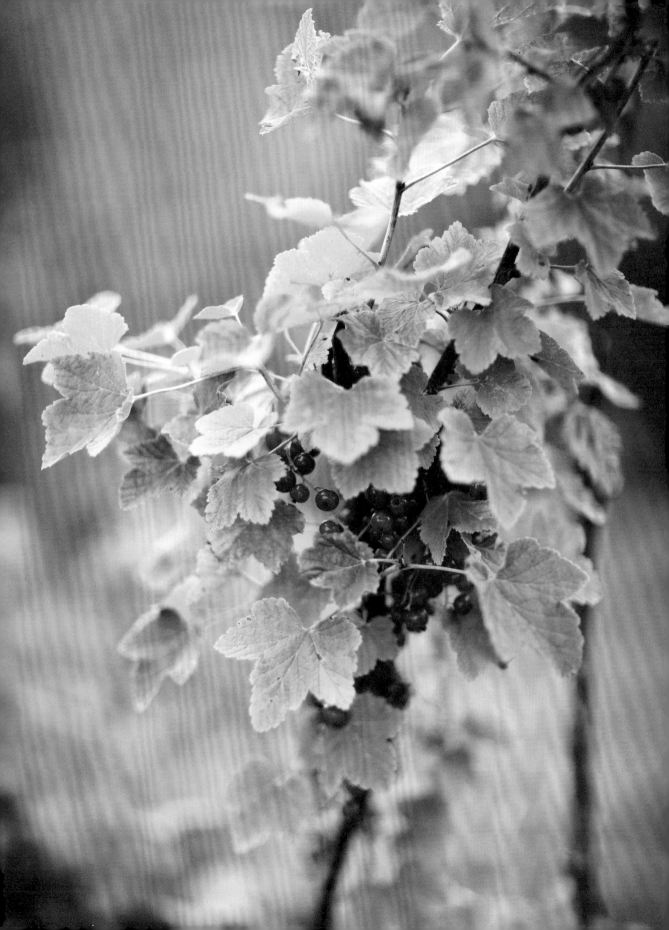

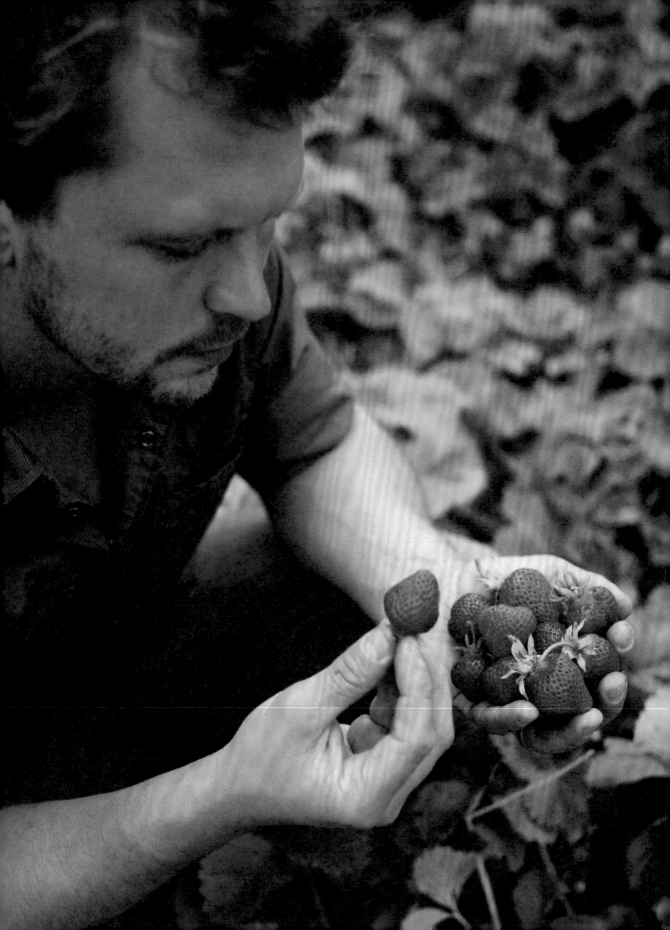

Currants

The three main types ('black', 'red' and 'white') are all extremely high in vitamin C. The bushes come in all shapes and sizes and many of the more compact varieties are ideally suited to growing in smaller spaces or even pots.

Harvesting can be tricky, in that you need to pull the currants off their 'strigs' using a dinner fork. Leave the fruits on the plant as long as possible to allow them to become sweeter, but if they are too bitter to eat raw they cook well and make superb cordials, jams and savoury jellies.

Gooseberry

Once this was a fixture in every cottage garden, but it seems to have fallen out of favour. This is a pity because it has a superb, rather aromatic quality, and if the fruit is allowed to ripen properly it can also be sweet enough to eat straight from the bush and to need little or no sugar when cooked. Another plus is that most varieties have needle-sharp thorns, making them ideal for inclusion in hedges (and if you have an established bush, you can supply the planting stock simply by popping cuttings from winter pruning in potting compost). In due course you will get plenty of mid-summer fruit – and if you don't want it, the local birds and voles will really benefit.

Plum

These don't seem particularly popular and so only one or two of the biggest varieties tend to appear in the shops.

However, there is a wide range of fruits available, varying from the smaller damsons and greengages to the heavy-cropping 'Victoria'. As well as making a great dessert fruit, many cook well – and of course across much of Europe they are fermented and distilled to make sliwowitz, rakia or eau de vie.

Raspberry

One of the great advantages of raspberries is that you can produce a huge crop from a relatively small space. A row of canes supported by wires will bear a heavy yield. These succulent fruits are the perfect way to introduce children to gardening and there is surely nothing more hedonistic than the joy of wandering along the row in the heat of high summer, popping sun-warmed fruit straight into the mouth. Eaten like this, there is no need for cream or sugar – but obviously it also cooks and preserves superbly well.

Strawberry

Few fruits can be as easy or quick to grow as a strawberry. This was originally a woodland plant, and one that reproduces by sending out straggling runners. Most strawberries have a comparatively short fruiting season, but you can extend this by planting early, mid- and late-fruiting varieties. They also do well in planters, making them ideal patio or balcony plants. Also, home-grown fruits always taste better, as most have a short shelf-life, so supermarkets tend to stock strains selected for longevity rather than flavour.

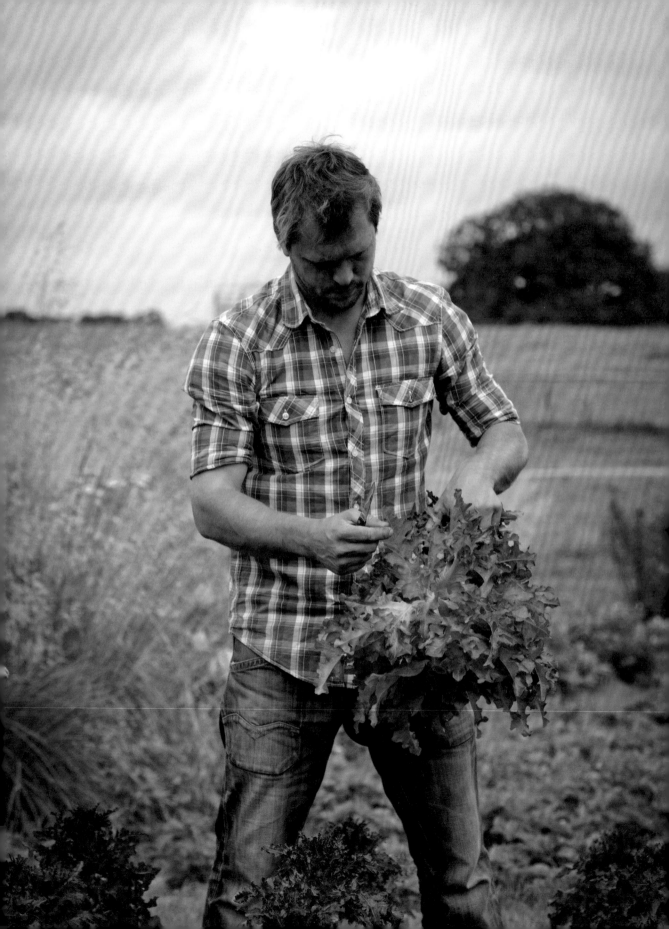

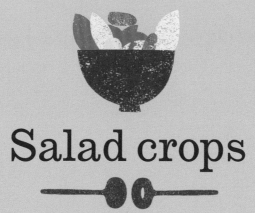

Salad crops

If you're looking for self-sufficiency with just one crop, salad is it. The plants take up little room and if you sow various varieties successively you could be picking leaves year round.

Salad has taken the country by storm in recent years, and now we expect a variety of colours, tastes and textures in our salad bowls, not just a limp lettuce leaf and a lonely slice or two of cucumber. In addition to a dozen varieties of lettuce, most supermarkets now stock a range of bagged leaves that contain blends of watercress, rocket and oriental greens.

Salad crops are easy to grow at home. They take up little space (you can grow them in seed trays on a windowsill) and they mature quicker than almost any other crop: three weeks from sowing to cutting. Many are suitable for 'cut-and-come-again' harvesting, allowing you to take three or four crops from one sowing over the course of the summer, which makes them very economical.

A fair number of varieties are also pretty hardy, which means they can be sown and harvested in the colder ends of the year, giving them one of the longest growing seasons of any crop. If you have a polytunnel or greenhouse to protect them from frost, you can provide yourself with salad leaves virtually all year round.

If you purchase a few different packs of seeds, you can experiment to create your own unique blend of varieties to suit your taste. A browse through any seed catalogue, printed or online, will reveal a bewildering range of salad varieties. Pak choi, iceberg and cos lettuces can supply 'crunch', while watercress, rocket and mizuma will give a peppery quality. Beetroot, lollo rosso and rainbow chard are just some of the coloured leaves that will give a dash of colour and a more robust background flavour to green salads.

If you're growing to sell, these mixed green leaves are a good bet, as they can be sold fairly easily, either in box schemes or direct to local hotels and restaurants. Alternatively, they can be liquidised to create 'power drinks', either for yourself or to feed the fast-growing health and fitness markets. Another possibility is to cook and liquidise them as baby foods.

Leaves have a very short shelf-life, though, so as well as creating an unusual mix of flavours with whatever value-added elements you can think of (e.g. packaging and dressings), freshness is absolutely key. If you are going to sell salad to consumers or businesses, you will probably need some form of chilled transport, and be aware that they need to be with the customer within 24 hours at the most.

Beetroot

For years the only way this member of the turnip family would appear on our plates was boiled or pickled and cold. It was a classic example of a vegetable that you either loved or hated.

Today we probably mostly eat beetroot grated into salad mixes or as baby leaves – although many people don't associate the name 'beet' leaves with the root vegetable. The leaves have a delicate flavour and the thin red stalks add a lovely splash of colour to a green salad. If you don't manage to pick the young leaves in time, you can still get a good root harvest off the plants later in the season.

Chicory

We normally encounter this slightly bitter leaf as a very pale 20cm torpedo on a greengrocer's shelf. These chicories will have been blanched by having the light excluded for a week or so, which increases sugar production and thus reduces the bitterness of the leaves. This process isn't strictly necessary, however, and the flavour of the heads when unforced adds a wonderful tang to salads, particularly if mixed with other leaves.

There are three main types of chicory available: witloof, sugarloaf and radicchio, with several varieties of each type. Radicchio is particularly interesting, as these develop a wonderful red colour as the thermometer dips in autumn, which gives an extra dash of colour to leaf mixes.

Corn salad

Also known as lamb's lettuce, these small succulent leaves have a distinctly sweet quality. They are very hardy and will grow throughout the winter – even tolerating frost – although they will slow down or even stop growing when conditions get very cold. They therefore do best with a little protection – a cloche or unheated greenhouse is normally enough to keep them going and provide clippings of fresh green leaves throughout the bleak winter months.

Endive

This curly, almost spikily-leafed plant is a mainstay of French salads, but has only recently started to become popular in salads over here.

Endive is hardy and so particularly valued for being available in late winter just when it is most difficult to find fresh produce for picking in the garden. Its

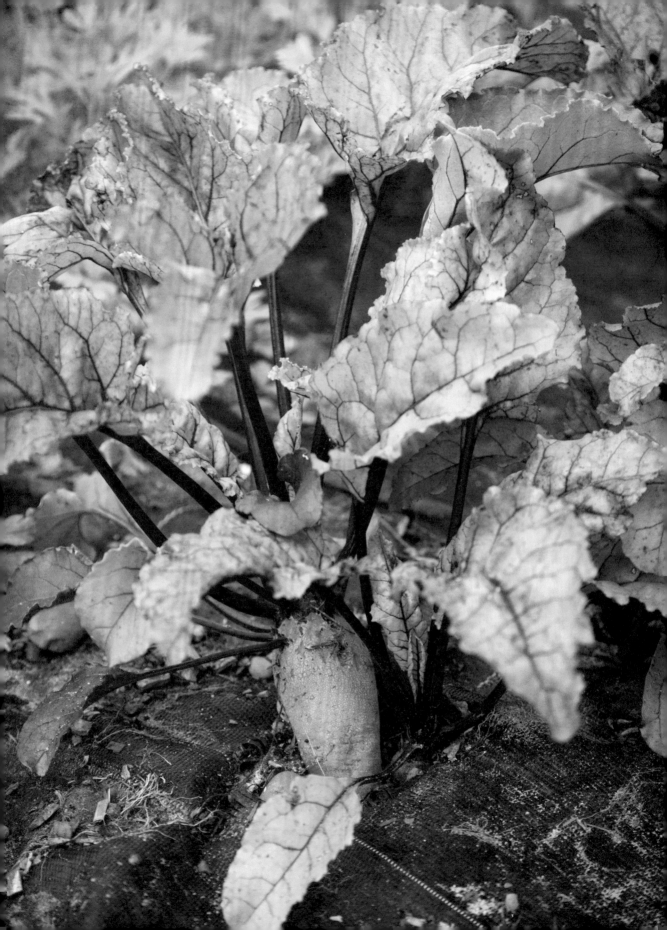

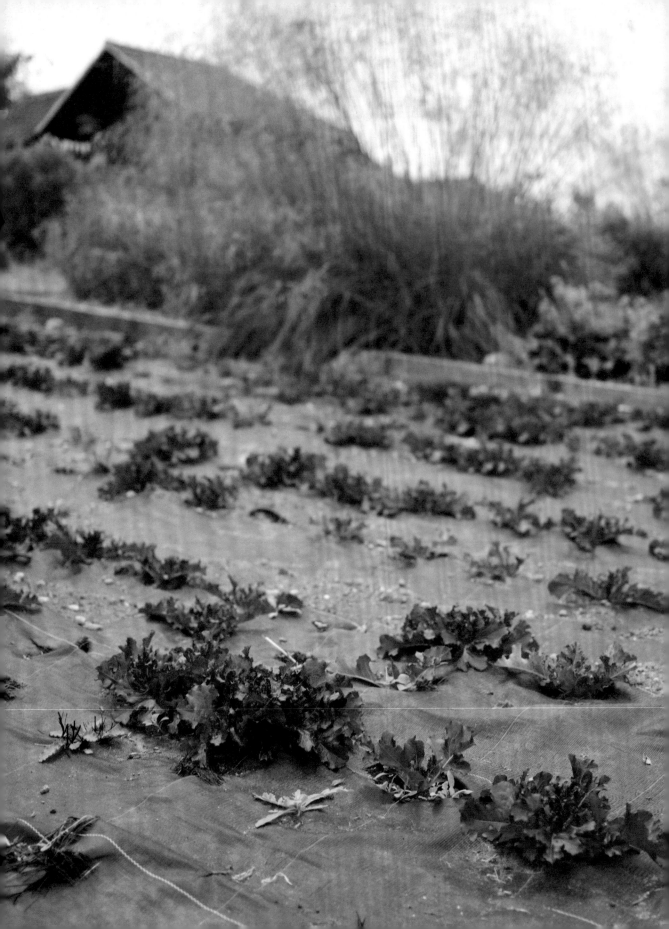

main drawback is that in its natural state it is bitter, but fortunately this is easy to overcome by blanching the leaves. All this means is depriving the plants of light – the simplest way being to place an upturned bucket over the plant a few days before harvesting.

Lettuces

There are simply dozens of this mainstay of the British green salad. This name might be the starting point, but lettuce doesn't have to be green. I always think a great salad should look and taste interesting, and to achieve that, colour, shape and texture are all critical.

There are some wonderfully colourful varieties available from seed suppliers (for example the brownish oak leaf and the rusty lollo rosso) and even within the green types there is a huge range of shades or those with coloured tints.

The texture and shape of lettuces also varies widely, so think about this too when choosing which lettuce you would like to grow. Generally lettuces are easy to grow (although they do need cool temperatures for germination) and are quick to mature, but they can bolt rapidly when the plant turns its attention from leaf to seed production or if temperatures become too hot. At that point it shoots up and the leaves become decidedly bitter. On the plus side, however, bolted lettuces can look attractive, resembling a Chinese pagoda, so if you don't mind disparaging comments from fellow allotment holders, you can leave them – otherwise the chickens will love them.

Pak choi

Until recently this was rarely seen anywhere other than Chinese restaurants, but it grows well here and when cut young it makes a succulent, crunchy addition to a mixed leaf salad.

If you leave the plants too long, the plants will develop a thick, bulbous stem that is delicious steamed or braised as a vegetable and is also great in stir-fries.

Rocket

I can never understand why it has taken the British so long to find out about this lovely peppery herb – nor can I work out why it is still so expensive. It grows like a weed, galloping away, and if you ever allow it to flower and run to seed, you will never need to plant it again – your beds will never be clear of it.

There are several varieties available which all have a similar flavour when home-grown, but wild rocket plants will usually last longer than other types.

Rocket grows happily outdoors from mid-spring to mid-autumn or indoors pretty much all year round.

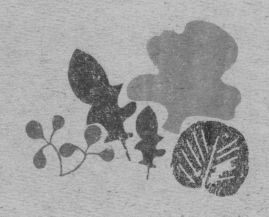

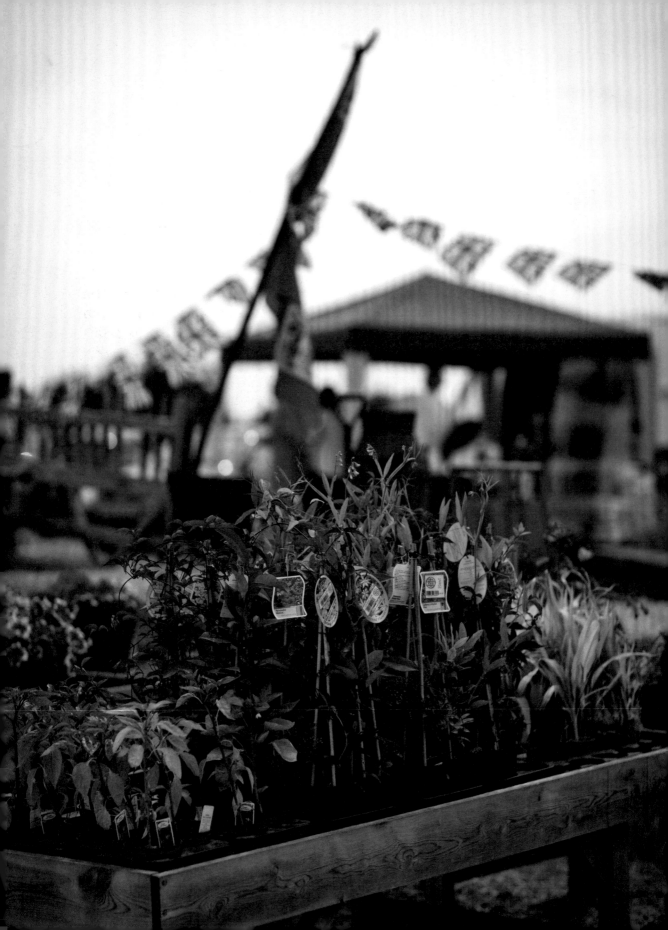

Rare vegetable and plant varieties

If you can't find a gap in the market for your veg, or the crops you want to grow are so cheap in the shops that it's not worth while growing them even for personal consumption, think about trying a few varieties you can't get elsewhere instead.

Although the supermarkets which supply some 75 per cent of the food we eat are getting more adventurous in their stocking policies, there are thousands of delicious and exciting vegetables that have yet to appear here – at least for sale in edible form. There are literally thousands of seeds available from specialist companies in this country and many more by mail order from overseas. Also, rather than buying ordinary souvenirs when overseas, if Customs allow it, why not bring back a pack of seeds instead? There are plenty of openings for the adventurous horticulturalist to produce interesting tastes, textures and scents, either for personal use or for sale to discerning customers.

Benefits

There are hundreds of delicious vegetables from around the world which are simply not available to buy. If you love food and experimentation in the kitchen, the only way you can get hold of many of these is to grow them yourself. And if you can find an interesting crop that people want to buy, yet which no one else can provide, the novelty justifies high prices if you decide to grow them as a business. For example, many modern chefs love to use unusual decoration around the plate: thus it was recently reported some upmarket London restaurants were paying £300 per kilo for hop shoots. An even more extreme example might be blueberries. Hailing from America, a decade ago they were almost unknown here, yet within a few years they have become one of our most popular soft fruits, almost eclipsing native white-, red- and blackcurrants.

Problems

While many unfamiliar crops are delicious, others are acquired tastes. Cultivating a completely new variety, let alone a new vegetable, is an experiment which will take at least a few months to bear fruit (no pun intended) and which still might prove a complete waste of time. Some will also need specialised cultivation techniques, and it's not always easy to get help and advice. Also, even when you do hit the jackpot, most potential customers are fairly conservative when it comes to a strange-looking leaf or root which they don't know how to cook, let alone what it tastes like.

Plants to try

Beginners would probably do best to avoid delicate plants such as okra or sweet potatoes, which come from the tropics. You can grow both here, but they aren't really suited to our climate and they will take up valuable greenhouse space and may have limited appeal. That said, if you are devoted to either and growing solely for yourself, then ignore this advice and add to your enjoyment of the meal with the knowledge you've grown it yourself.

Celeriac

Although this swollen-root version of the blanched leaves and stalks of its familiar relative are popular on the Continent, it never seems to have caught on here. This is a pity because in many ways it is more versatile. It roasts, mashes and steams well and it arguably has a better flavour – one with a distinctly nutty edge.

Celeriac is relatively easy to grow, but you will have to start early in the year from seed because it rarely features in garden centres as young plants. It needs occasional hoeing and watering in dry weather, but it is fairly pest- and disease-resistant. Its biggest drawback is that it is very slow-growing. Even if you get the seedlings into the ground by Easter, they will most likely not be ready to harvest until late autumn.

Chillies

If any one plant has burst into British cuisine more explosively than any other, surely the chilli would take the prize? Most of those on sale are 'jalapenos', but there are hundreds of varieties available from specialist suppliers in every conceivable shape, colour and – of course – heat. I particularly like the brightly coloured little round ones which stand up, rather than hang down, from the plant.

They are very easy to grow and many can be very attractive, so although they are very frost-sensitive, if you grow them in pots and bring these inside, they make a decorative Christmas ornament.

It goes without saying they work extremely well in combination with other produce – and this is also a great way of harnessing the late summer glut for the long winter and spring. In their own right they make a great relish when combined with other vegetables to make chutneys, pickles, relishes and sauces. Chillies naturally lend themselves to flavouring oil, vinegars and jellies.

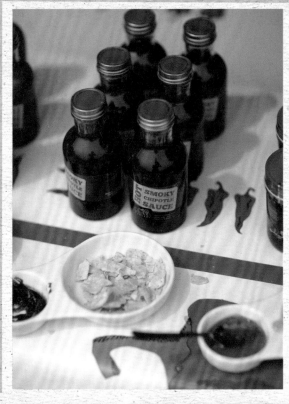

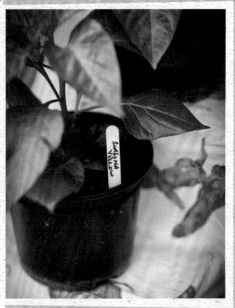

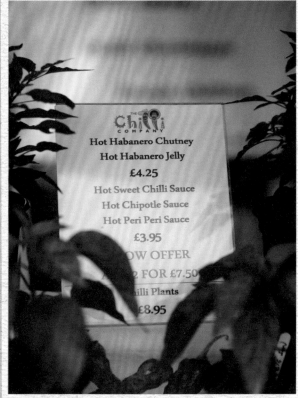

The Chilli COMPANY

Hot Habanero Chutney
Hot Habanero Jelly
£4.25
Hot Sweet Chilli Sauce
Hot Chipotle Sauce
Hot Peri Peri Sauce
£3.95
OW OFFER
2 FOR £7.50
hilli Plants
£8.95

If any ONE PLANT has BURST
into the BRITISH Cuisine
more EXPLOSIVELY than any
OTHER, surely the CHILLI
would take the PRIZE?

They can also look wonderful bottled whole, particularly if you use a mix of unusual colours and shapes.

Chinese broccoli
This is a sort of cross between asparagus and broccoli and has the advantage of the best qualities of each. In other words it has a fantastic flavour, yet is easy and quick to grow. It steams and stir fries very well and seems likely to become more popular over the coming years.

Hamburg parsley
This looks a bit like a thin parsnip, and while popular on the Continent it is rarely grown here. It is a versatile vegetable; both the root and parsley-like leaves can be eaten. The tubers have a flavour reminiscent of a parsnip crossed with celery while the leaves live up to the name. It is easy to grow in a shady spot – sow around Easter, ideally in ground that has been warmed by black plastic covering. The first roots can be lifted in late autumn or left in the soil until required during the winter. For an interesting twist, try slicing thinly and deep-frying to make crisps or chips.

Kohl rabi
This looks a bit like a turnip with leaves sprouting from the sides, but it is actually a swollen stem. It is grown extensively across Europe, but has never really caught on here – a pity because it does better than many other root vegetables in shallow soils. It only takes a couple of months from sowing to harvest, which makes it an interesting option in small gardens. Better still, it is a versatile vegetable which can both be steamed or grated raw and added to salads.

Salsify (scorzonera)
This root vegetable is readily available but seems rarely grown and is even rarer in supermarkets and greengrocers. It looks like a rather emaciated parsnip, but tastes completely different. Some people compare the flavour to that of oysters and certainly it is delicious when steamed and dressed with butter, vinaigrette or a lightly scented herb oil.

Seed sprouts
Many oriental cuisines make heavy use of the sweet, tender young shoots that emerge from energy-rich beans and seeds. Apart from appearing in salads and in spring rolls, they don't really feature in the British diet. They should, because they are perfect for cultivation in even the smallest flat, growing quickly and year-round, so sowings in a cupboard or on a windowsill every few days will produce enough seedlings to satisfy a small family.

There are two broad ways of cultivating these. The first is to place seeds such as adzuki, mung, alfalfa and fenugreek in a jar, cover with water for an hour, pour it off, fasten a piece of muslin over the top with an elastic band and rinse with fresh water twice a day. Then grow on in the dark until ready. Alternatively, plants like mustard and cress can be grown on blotting paper in a tray on a windowsill and harvested with a pair of scissors to scatter in sandwiches and salads.

A GROWING BUSINESS?

The British have long been keen gardeners, but thanks to the plethora of gardening programmes and press articles this interest has exploded over recent years. Anyone with green fingers can potentially cash in on this by growing unusual plants from seeds and cuttings, but many people lack the time, effort and foresight to do this for themselves. Instead they impulse buy at the garden centre or supermarket. These may sell trays of bedding plants at a price you could never hope to match, but the range is usually remarkably restricted. This opens up the possibility of supplying a local market with slightly quirkier varieties. This works particularly well if you have established plants. Soft fruit needs to be pruned – so why not pop the cuttings in a pot of compost instead of throwing them away? Strawberries don't breed true from seed; in the wild they reproduce mainly by sending out runners along the ground to root a few feet away – simply peg these into a little tub of compost and a few weeks later you have a new plant to sell or give away. Globe artichokes are another great example – their roots need regular separation to keep the parent plant healthy, so why not pot these up too?

✔ ADVANTAGES

Growing seedlings is very flexible and doesn't require much space. You can do this in yoghurt pots ranged along a flat windowsill, although a greenhouse is much better. Because the young plants are, by definition, small, they don't take up much space. There is also generally a very quick turnaround – tomato or chilli seeds planted in February are ready for planting out in April. This sort of eight-week start-to-finish cycle means you can be very adaptable, growing successions of different seeds according to local demand and the season. And at the very least, because almost all seed suppliers give you more than you need for personal use, rather than trying to store one year's excess for the next, you can recoup the cost of the packet by selling the surplus – or at least giving them away as gifts to friends.

✔ DISADVANTAGES

By far the biggest problem is the intense competition from garden centres, supermarkets and online suppliers which rely heavily on imports from vast greenhouses in warmer parts of the world where labour is cheaper. Unless you branch out into the unusual, both you and any theoretical customers will save a great deal of time, effort and money buying direct from the big boys.

Also, owing to their size, seedlings are very vulnerable to pests like slugs and voles. One momentary lapse of attention and the entire crop can be devastated. Just as bad, because the pots and plants are so small, they can dry out quickly – a weekend without water in a centrally heated flat and you could lose the lot.

CASE STUDY

'The SECRET of building a successful farm business is NOT to SPECIALISE or DIVERSIFY, but to do BOTH SIMULTANEOUSLY.' Explains the Chilli Company's Adrian Nuttall.

Born in Nairobi, the son of RAF parents, Adrian grew up with spicy food, but found it difficult to get hold of chillies in England. Adrian's personal epiphany started on a stag night in 1995 when he had a tipsy argument with a chef about whether chillies would grow here. 'It stayed with me and the next day I got hold of a couple of chillies and planted the seeds,' he explains. 'Two or three germinated and I grew them in pots on the windowsill – if I hadn't had that argument and if the seeds hadn't worked, I would probably have never pursued it, let alone built a successful business around them.'

The plants thrived in the warmth and light of his windowsill; however, they produced far too many fruits for him and his wife, Denise, to consume fresh. The couple were soon making a variety of sauces, curries and jams to use the surplus. This naturally led to requests from family and friends and then, 11 years ago, he began to take his stock to farmers' markets. The business was still no more than a weekend sideline (albeit having progressed from windowsill to conservatory to greenhouse).

A few years later, and now with two children, the chillies had progressed into a busy sideline, but Adrian was still travelling a lot on business. 'In 2002 Denise turned to me and said, "Do you realise you've been away for half of your daughter's life?" I knew I had to do something radical, and apart from computerising payrolls, growing chillies was my only other area of expertise,' he laughs. His day job as an

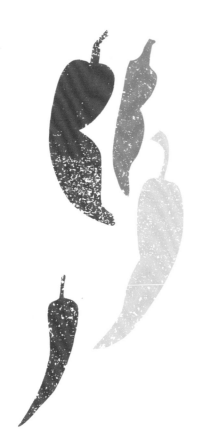

IT consultant took the couple and their young family to France for a year in 2005. When they returned home they decided to go into chilli growing on a large scale. The couple found an old nursery near Mendlesham, in Suffolk. 'It had five polytunnels, two greenhouses, 10 stables, a couple of ponds, a cart lodge and a derelict barn,' he says. 'We moved in at Christmas 2005, and at the beginning of 2006 we filled one greenhouse with seedlings, then got to work re-covering the polytunnels and renovating the main barn, which we opened as a Mexican restaurant.'

It hasn't been plain sailing; in 2008 the recession saw the restaurant struggle, but more importantly Adrian realised that even though he was within a stone's throw of home he wasn't getting into bed until well after midnight. So now it is a less formal café open only during the day.

Deprived of the restaurant income, the couple returned to their original idea of creating sauces and jams which they have since persuaded delis, farm shops, Adnams, Fortnum & Mason and Bentalls, in Kingston-upon-Thames, to stock. In addition the couple have opened a farm shop next to the café, which stocks local eggs, vegetables and other traditional farm shop produce. It was at this point that Adrian approached me to make a chilli sausage – and it flew off the counter. His next step is to invest in a smoker so he can sell a new range of products, such as cheese coated in chilli and lightly smoked.

Adrian says no one knows how many varieties of chillies there are because many have different names in different countries, but estimates put it at 2,000–8,000. The Nuttalls grow around 50 varieties, planting most as seeds in January, but overwinter one or two inside. In general, however, the cost of keeping the greenhouse frost-free with oil-fired heaters makes this prohibitive on a big scale. 'That said, we also generally end up with a plant in a corner somewhere which gets woody and pot-bound and ends up as a rather attractive stunted bush.'

In addition to fruiting plants and those for sale, they grow 50 or so more varieties, partly for a colourful display for visitors, but also to experiment with in the kitchen, 'If something works well, we grow it the following year on a large scale.'

Over the years he says it has been easy to see how the appeal of each variety breaks down into a clear demographic pattern. 'Every time you see a group of 18–30 males, you know they are going to head for the hottest,' he laughs. 'Then you get older customers who've done a bit of travelling who want to recreate a certain flavour or experience they've come across in their journeys. Then you get ladies who want something ornamental, but that produces something they can cook with.'

Adrian is convinced that there is far more to a chilli's appeal than just heat. 'One green chilli has more vitamin C than five oranges and it lowers blood pressure and cholesterol while increasing libido and stimulating the release of endorphins – the chemicals that cause the sensation of happiness in the brain,' he says. 'I wouldn't say they are a superfood, but we've only scratched the surface of their potential.'

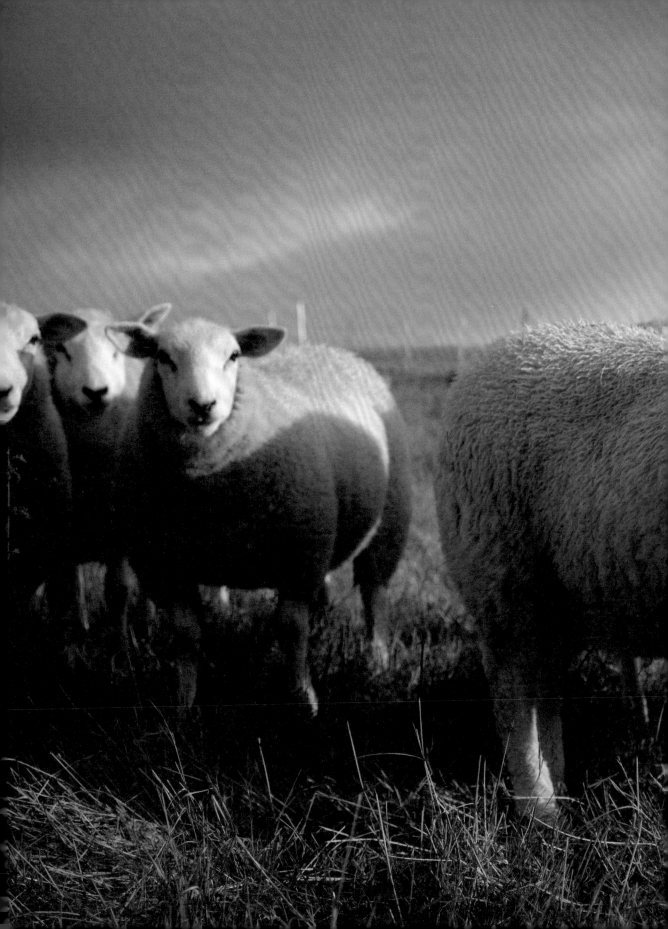

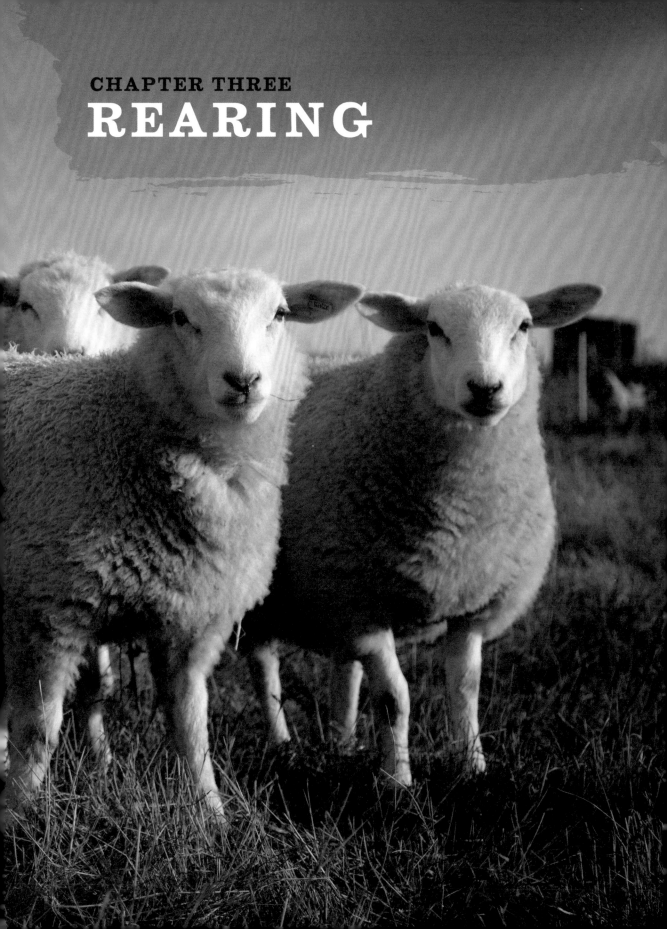

REARING

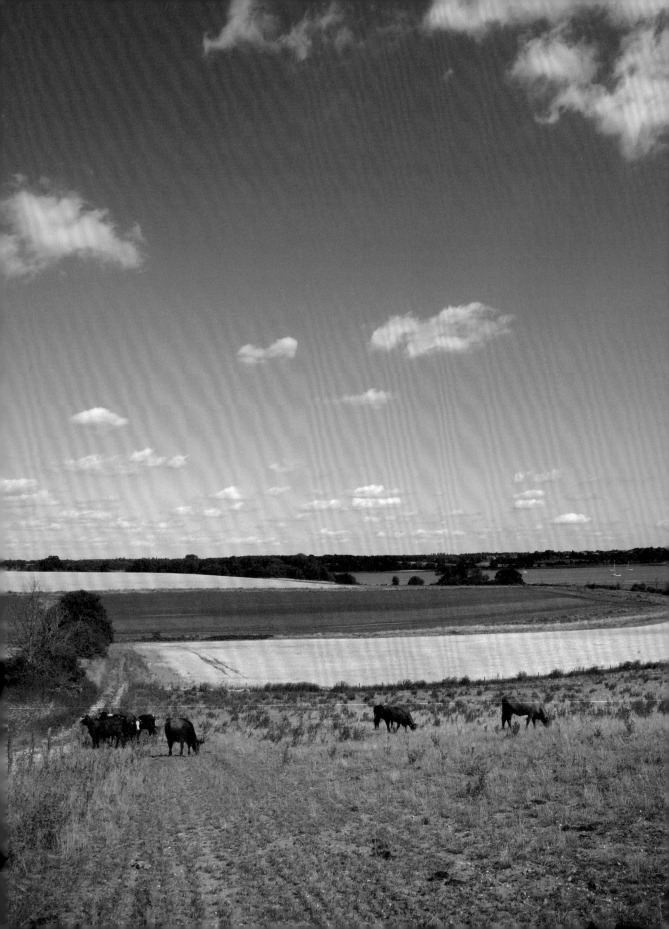

MY PIGS AND OTHER ANIMALS

RAISING LIVESTOCK

To my mind livestock are a critical part of farming. Animals are part of the natural cycle of life and in an ideal world I feel they should be an integral part of any food production. I love growing my own vegetables, but however satisfying it is to persuade a seemingly inert and lifeless seed into a bushy and productive courgette or chilli plant, you just can't have a relationship with it. Even those people who are convinced that talking to plants or playing them music boosts yields would have to concede they are never going to come skipping up to you with joy in their hearts, let alone chat back.

It was pigs that hooked me into farming. As I've already explained, I just love them for their personalities – but I am realistic. From the outset the bulk of all my animals are destined for dinner plates. As a carnivore myself I have no problem with this, provided I know I am giving them happy, freedom-filled lives, and in return I get so much enjoyment from them – whether it's chilling out watching the cattle slowly chewing the cud in the evening sunshine, seeing gangs of spring lambs tearing round the fields like out-of-control teenagers, or scratching a favourite sow behind the ears as she tucks into her breakfast.

There is no reason why you shouldn't share this enjoyment, wherever you live, but it doesn't mean to say you have to be a meat eater to include animals in your plans. It is perfectly possible to enjoy animal husbandry while producing pedigree breeding stock for others. Generating eggs and milk doesn't directly involve death either (although in the process of rearing these livestock there will be born some unwanted, unproductive male offspring which will inevitably need to be culled at some point). Bees are even better for the scrupulous as there is no killing required – although I suppose a supreme moralist might say apiarists are exploiting the industrious little creatures by stealing their surplus production.

Keeping any kind of livestock involves a moral responsibility. If you don't water a plant and it withers, it's a pity; do the same to a pig or chicken and it's unforgivable (not to mention making you liable to prosecution). For the same reasons, before buying any livestock you need to plan everything carefully. It is easy to buy young poultry on impulse at a market without having suitable housing waiting at home. It is much more easy to think you have prepared the ground by sorting out fencing, feeders and so on, yet to have failed to work out how you are going to use the produce and whether or not you want to go on to sell it. One common omission, for example, is to research where you can slaughter small batches of unusual animals (for example, many abattoirs won't

handle pigs at all and those that do may not be happy with more hairy traditional breeds, let alone a wild boar).

These are only considerations to take into account, however, and they should not put you off if you're really keen on the idea. Breeding, rearing and tending animals is incredibly rewarding – indeed it can be seriously addictive. Nor does it always require large amounts of land. Of course you can't really keep a cow in a Surbiton garden like Tom and Barbara Good did, but you can certainly have a few hens (or, better still, bantams, which are just a scaled-down version). If you do have a little more land than this then keeping goats, sheep or even pigs becomes possible. And even if you have no more than a top-floor flat, bees are still a possibility – so perhaps we should start with these, rather than my beloved pigs…

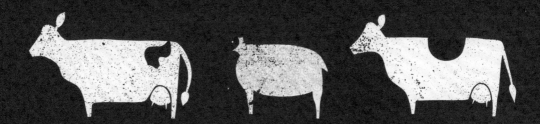

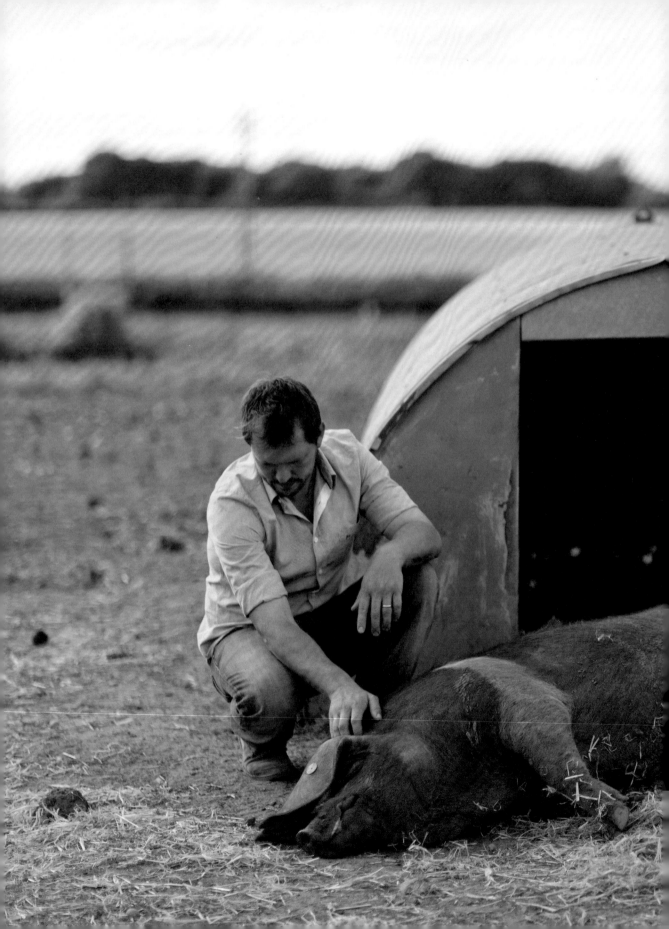

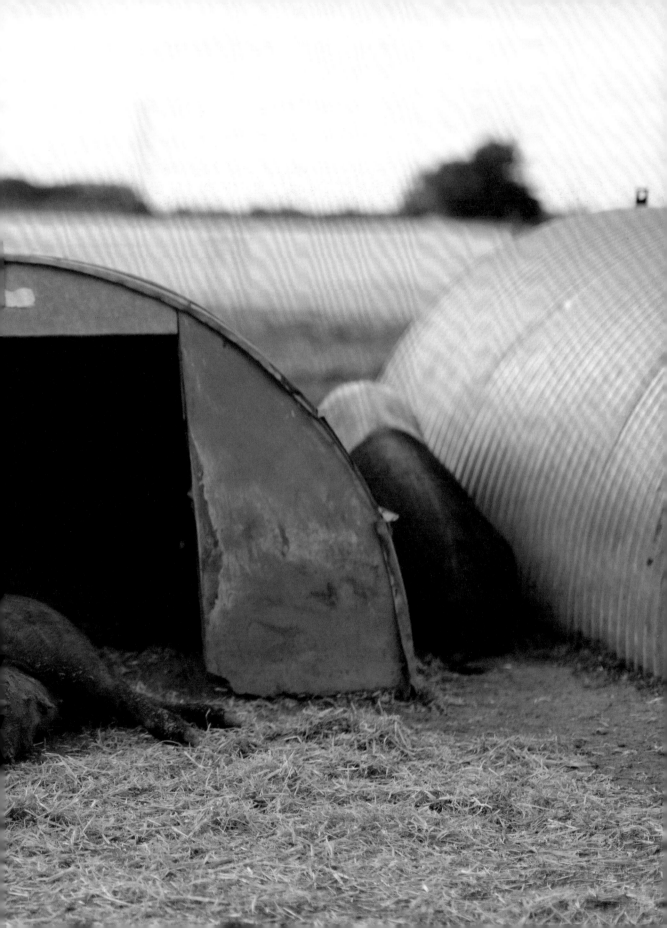

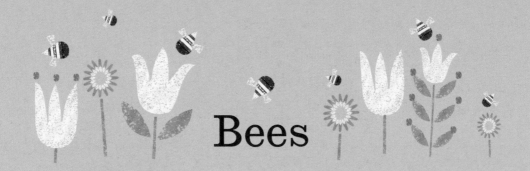

Bees

Bees buzzing in and out of flowers on a sunny day epitomises a British summer. It might not occur to you to keep them; however, these dual-purpose insects will not only pollinate your crops but leave you delicious honey at the end.

Many people have an innate fear of bees, which is all too often rooted in an unfortunate childhood encounter. This is a pity because bees can be the perfect starting point for someone with little experience of gardening or rearing but who likes the idea of producing their own food. Even better, they are ideal for anyone with little or no land.

Indeed, some of the most productive hives in Britain are mounted on flat city roofs where, in a good year, each one can yield up to 60kg of honey and about 3.5kg of wax. Alternatively, farmers are often only too delighted to have a couple of hives in the corner of a field in return for their occupants' pollination services.

The hives themselves are fairly cheap – particularly if you buy a flat-pack self-assembly kit – and in addition the only essential equipment you need is some protective clothing. This looks terrifying, like something from *The Andromeda Strain*, but actually it is little more than a veil, boiler suit and gloves. The amount of time and labour spent is up to you.

Apart from an occasional inspection, the colony will pretty much look after itself, although many apiarists find dealing with the hive very therapeutic and will create any excuse to potter with their bees.

Benefits

Bee colonies need virtually no space to produce large quantities of honey and wax every autumn. The former is not only a natural sweetener, but it also has a wide range of health-giving properties and a very long shelf-life (it never goes off). The wax produced can be processed into candles and polishes or used in a wide range of crafts (for example, batik).

Problems

An ever-changing variety of pests and diseases are undoubtedly the biggest headache for the modern beekeeper. A century ago almost all of Britain's

ADVANTAGES

Crop POLLINATORS
NEED little space / EQUIPMENT
NEED little TIME / LABOUR

DISADVANTAGES

DISEASES
OPPOSition from
NEIGHBOURS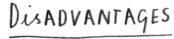
CHEAP Honey
IMPORTS
available

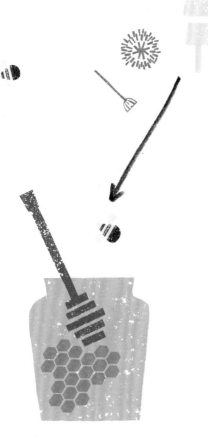

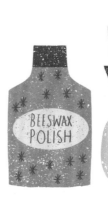

BEESWAX POLISH

SOAP

colonies of the native black bee were wiped out by Isle of Wight disease, which was caused by a combination of a parasitic mite, viral infection and stress from overcrowding. The solution was found by Brother Adam of Buckfast Abbey, in Devon, who used naturally resistant Italian bees to create a new strain of docile yellow bees, which bear the Abbey's name to this day. However, bacterial infections such as foulbrood remain a constant problem. Then in the 1990s a fresh plague arrived in the form of varroa: a tiny blood-sucking parasite which is relatively harmless to its natural Asian bee hosts, but which was anything but to European strains. It can be treated with minute quantities of insecticide, but if ignored yields will fall and eventually the hive will die. The most recent problem of all, Colony Collapse Disorder (CCD), is causing consternation in the United States, where it causes apparently healthy hives to fail completely.

Resistance from neighbours can be a problem, too. Although domesticated bees are normally very docile, many people – particularly parents with young children – can be alarmed by their presence. Siting the hives so the insects' flight paths avoid humans is one solution – for example, if you place the colony next to a tall hedge, where it is largely invisible, the bees will have to fly in over the neighbour's garden above head height. Another solution is simply not to tell them – they will probably never know, although it might be responsible to enquire discreetly about any serious insect allergies that they might have.

Produce

As I've already said, the two obvious products of your hive will be honey and wax, with wax offering other produce from its usage, such as polish or candles. If you want to sell your produce, there is always a ready market for honey, although there are plenty of cheap imports available in the shops. Unless you have several hives and are producing huge numbers of jars, you can probably sell most of your honey to friends through word of mouth, but otherwise many health-food shops will be only too delighted to stock a locally produced honey.

If you want to use the wax to make candles, this can be great fun and gives you the opportunity to create something truly unique and marketable as craft goods. (See the next page for information on candle-making.)

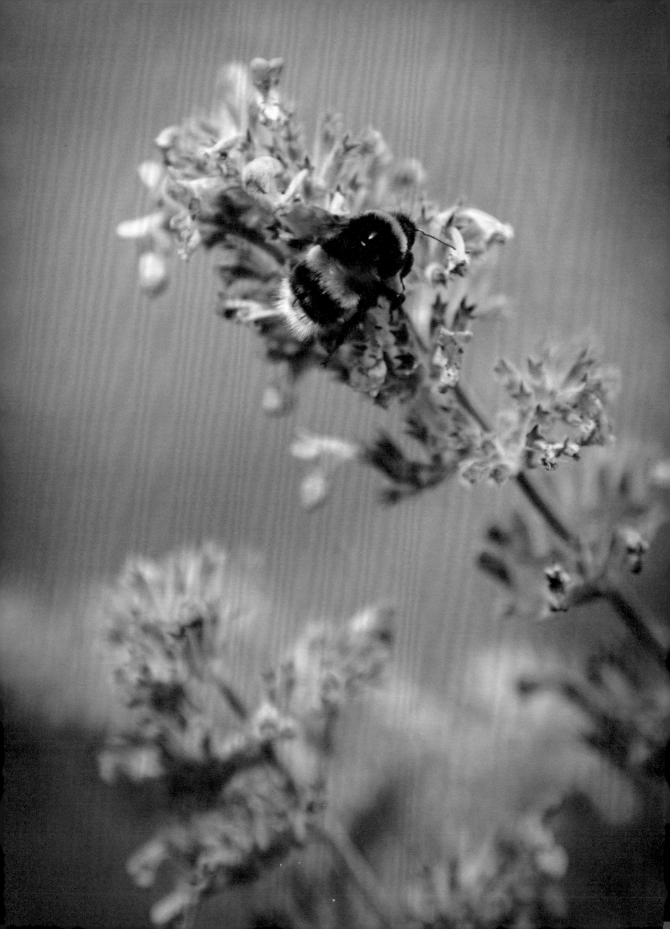

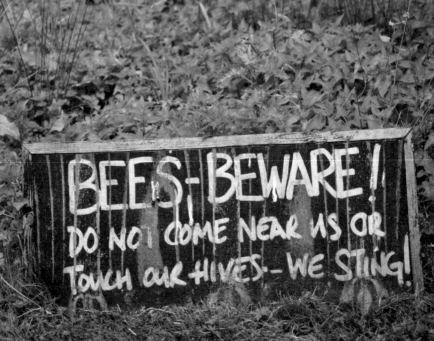

BEAUTIFUL BEESWAX CANDLES

Beeswax candles have long been prized for their superior light, longevity and lack of smoke. Today most commercial candles are made from paraffin wax, however, so there is potentially a great market for high-quality handmade candles.

Beeswax melts at 62–64°C and this is best done in a pan in a water bath (the wax mustn't come into direct contact with the heat or water). Use a sugar thermometer to check the temperature. It is vital to use really pure wax for the best results, although you can dye this with a range of natural substances or incorporate scents or herbs to create a unique result. The wick is vital to the final product because it is up this that the molten wax is drawn by capillary action to reach the flame. If it is too thin for the candle's diameter excess wax will flow down the outside of the candle and the pool which forms beneath the flame may even extinguish it. If it is too thick, however, it is the wick rather than the wax which burns, producing a very smoky flame. A beeswax candle requires a much thicker wick than its paraffin equivalent. There are four basic techniques of candle making:

✔ POURING

This is the way to make the longest candles. Molten wax, just above the melting point, is dribbled down a wick into a reservoir. As it runs down the wick it solidifies in a thin layer along the string. The process is repeated and every three or four times the still-soft candle is rolled along a worktop to ensure it is straight. When the desired diameter is reached, the icicle of wax at the end is removed with a warm knife and the candle is left to air-cool.

✔ MOULDED

These are probably the easiest candles to make. Specialist craft suppliers sell a wide variety of moulds. Some come in one piece and require a release agent, which can give variable results, but the easiest are made of silicon and have a slit along one side to allow easy removal of the candle. The wick is threaded through a hole in the bottom (the candle is moulded upside down) and held taut at what will eventually be its base with two sticks.

✔ DIPPING

This is easier than pouring but essentially uses the same principles of allowing the wax to solidify in layers along the wick. A length of wick is folded in half and the double ends are lowered into the molten wax. Temperature is critical to both dipping and pouring – at 77°C it forms thin smooth layers, but at around 70°C these are thicker. Generally both processes start and finish with warmer wax to give a uniform finish but use cooler wax in the middle to speed things up.

✔ ROLLED

It is easy to make attractive candles using the sheets of moulded foundation wax which would normally form the basis of the combs. Soften these slightly in a water bath (obviously without reaching melting point), then place the wick along one edge and roll gently.

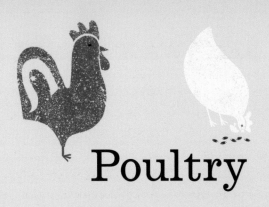

Poultry

When most people think of keeping animals for food production, particularly in gardens or small urban spaces, the humble chicken is often the first animal to come to mind, but there are other fowl that can be just as rewarding to rear.

Man has domesticated birds for their meat and eggs for thousands of years and they are still an important source of food today. Most are particularly good for small-scale farming because they are quick-growing and need little space or specialist attention. It is also one area where it is very easy to be totally self-sufficient in at least one product: three or four hens will lay more eggs than most families consume. Alternatively, the quality of your own genuinely free-range roasting fowl will be infinitely better than anything you can buy in the shops.

Poultry are also inexpensive to buy and keep. Indeed, you can get ex-commercial laying hens almost free, because as the birds age they begin to lay fewer, but larger, eggs. These are still perfectly edible, but the economics of commercial egg production are delicately balanced and fewer larger eggs tips the equation into a loss for the big farmers – who supply 98 per cent of the 11 billion eggs we consume in Britain every year. As a result most farmers cull their laying flocks at 18 months, so they will happily sell the 'spent' birds for a few pence each. Or you might want to think of something more unusual. Quail lay beautiful mottled eggs, for example, while some strains of duck are almost as prolific as commercial hens, producing a constant supply of big rich eggs that are worth three or four times as much as the hen equivalent. Even at the top end of the price range, a pedigree goose from a show-winning strain is rarely worth more than £100, so setting yourself up with a small flock is much cheaper than buying most other livestock.

These birds are also generally hardy (except quail), so apart from the occasional dose of wormer in their water, your vet's bills should be negligible. (To be brutally honest, sick birds are generally knocked on the head rather than being medicated.) Poultry will also find a lot of their own food if given the opportunity to – much of it as insect pests – and they can also be engaging, many having distinct characters that can be great fun in the garden or farmyard.

On the downside, however, if you are intending to rear birds as a business, you should note that as poultry is such a mainstay of modern diets it is a very competitive market (this is particularly true when it comes to hens), which can make it very difficult to find a niche. One of the biggest problems of production for market is processing. Even on the smallest of backyard scales, the guts, which are smelly and a magnet for rats, can pose awkward disposal problems. For most people, however, plucking is a bigger headache. Most mammalian livestock can simply be skinned in a couple of minutes. You can do this with birds, but most customers expect their chicken or turkey to come with its feathers removed but skin intact. This is even more vital when it comes to geese (after all it is the pints of rich fat which ooze from this which make it such a luxury food). However, birds are covered with at least three types of feathers and it can take many laborious minutes to dress just one goose, let alone your Christmas output. Of course, there are machines which will do the job and you could use the ultimate in 'Brazilians' – dipping them in a mix of scalding water and wax before peeling off the fluffy covering. Perhaps the simplest solution, though, is to persuade a specialised local abattoir to handle your birds for you.

Another disadvantage is that these birds are magnets for unwanted visitors. Foxes and badgers will readily snatch your precious poultry (they seem to have an unerring talent for grabbing your favourite). Worse, if a predator gets in among a confined flock the panicking birds can trigger a killing spree which can cost you dozens of birds in a matter of minutes. So you do need to lock them away every night and may also need to provide protection during the day. Even less welcome will be the rats which will inevitably arrive to pick up spilled food and to grab the occasional chick.

One of the great advantages of keeping poultry is that there really is a bird or breed to fit almost every situation. If you have plenty of space turkeys can be great fun, with the stags from some of the rarer breeds making for a striking addition to the garden's appearance. Geese also double up as great lawnmowers (although they come with an attendant pollution problem which makes them unsuitable for tidy gardeners and families with toddlers. At the other end of the spectrum, you can keep quail in a small aviary (or even a hutch).However, it is probably sensible to start with the most practical all-rounder: the chicken.

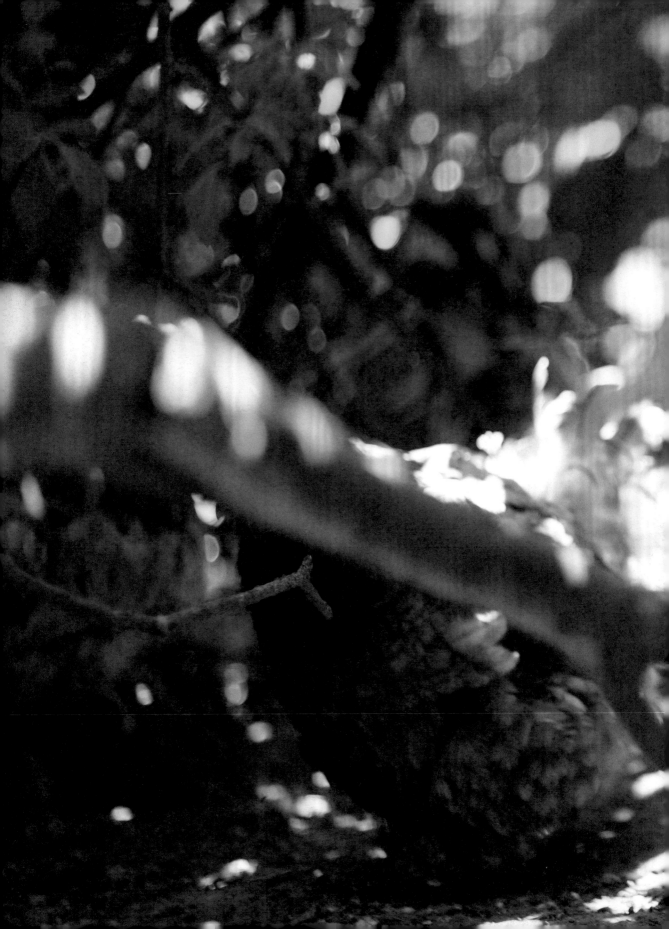

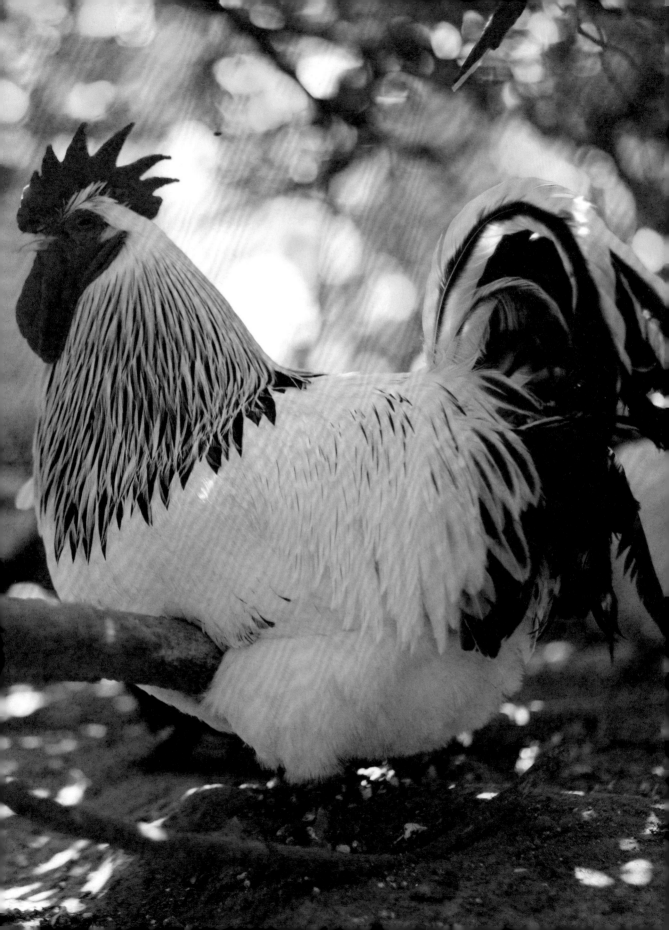

Chickens

Chickens are descended from Asian jungle fowl, which live in the forest in ordered family groups. Domesticated poultry have a similar social structure, with each bird occupying its own niche in the hierarchy (this is where we get the phrase 'pecking order'). As a result, you can spend hours simply studying the various personalities as the flock forage across the lawn or work their way through the vegetable patch. They also, obviously, produce two great foods – eggs and meat – that have been a vital part in human diets around the world since the dawn of time.

Housing

After several millennia in captivity, chickens and in particular bantams (literally scaled-down versions) are very happy in a remarkably small space. Battery chickens used to be kept at a density of four birds to a half-metre-square cage. These are now banned, thankfully, but their commercial 'free range' replacements are still kept at the same densities at night – although at least they are free to move around the crowded shed.

You will want to give them much more room than this, of course. The nicest way of all is to have a nocturnal shed to protect them from foxes which is also fitted with nest boxes to make egg collection easy. Once they are used to this as 'home' you let them out to wander at will, knowing they will return under their own steam at dusk. This is often unrealistic in towns, however, where the best solution is those moveable arks where the sleeping quarters are housed above or at the end of a wire netting run. Ready-made runs such as the 'Eglu' allow about half a square metre per bird, so make that a bare minimum if you build your own.

Although in many ways hens are low maintenance, they do need protection from inclement weather and predators at night and they also produce a lot of manure while roosting. Conventional housing has the drawback that it is often pretty stationary, meaning the birds peck around the same basic area; but I had a brainwave of getting an old caravan, knocking out the floor and replacing it with slats wide enough to let the droppings fall through while still keeping foxes out. I reasoned that if we left the wheels on the caravan, we could move it every few days to give the birds fresh ground while minimising cleaning and preventing the soil under the roosts getting too scorched by the fresh droppings.

Feed

Whether you are rearing chickens for eggs or meat, for personal consumption or sale, quality is going to be key. You want something that is clearly superior

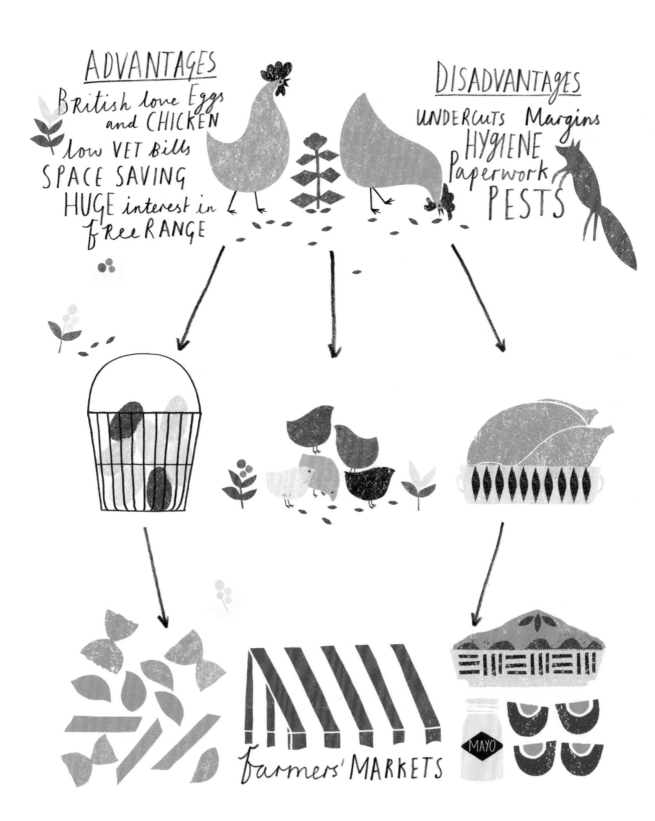

ADVANTAGES
British love Eggs
and CHICKEN
low VET Bills
SPACE SAVING
HUGE interest in
Free RANGE

DISADVANTAGES
UNDERcuts Margins
HYGIENE
Paperwork
PESTS

MAYO

Farmers' MARKETS

to the birds you find in the shops and this is going to be largely dictated by their diet. Many people forget that chickens are omnivores and think they will lay happily with just a few handfuls of corn every day. In fact both egg and meat production require plenty of protein, so they positively tend towards the carnivorous end of the spectrum. If you watch them closely as they forage and scratch across the lawn (and chicken watching can becomes seriously addictive), you will see they are scouring the grass for bugs and worms which they pounce on with all the ferocity of their velociraptor ancestors. Indeed, I have even seen a whole, living, mouse disappear down one's beak. In other words, they crave and need plenty of high-protein food.

The simplest solution is to buy sacks of ready-mixed 'layers' or 'growers' pellets. These contain just the right balance of nutrients, carbohydrates and protein. Unfortunately the last of this usually comes from imported soya or fish meal, this can cause problems as a producer for a niche market you may want to steer clear of GM. However, a high percentage of soya grown globally now tends to be genetically modified, while fish meal has all sorts of environmental issues.

Actually, on a backyard scale you may not need to buy in any food at all. If your birds are allowed to forage for themselves they will find most of what they need – particularly in summer. Chickens are natural hunters, loving nothing more than to peck and scratch, gobbling up anything that moves. If you let your birds roam freely across allotments, your veg garden or fresh pasture you can turn this to your advantage, using them as natural pest controllers. They are at their best when allowed to wander beneath fruit trees and shrubs as they will clean up pests such as caterpillars, sawfly larvae and leather jackets. It has to be said, though, that a lot of big meat chickens wandering across the vegetable patch can also do a fair amount of damage to your crops, so keep watch and be prepared to step in quickly if things start to go awry!

The other great source of food comes from kitchen scraps (unlike pigs, it is legal to feed household scraps to poultry). Meat waste shouldn't go onto the compost heap because it will attract flies, rats and foxes, but almost all will disappear down a chicken (for obvious reasons you will want to avoid feeding them chicken, although they are extremely cannibalistic and will certainly eat poultry if given a chance).

Another solution is to grow your own food for your birds. Soya may have a particularly high protein content, but other legumes can provide this too. Broad beans and peas grow well in Britain, for example, and another idea is to follow the French example and feed a high proportion of maize which, as well as adding to the eating quality, turns the skin and subcutaneous fat yellow. Until recently supermarkets were adamant British consumers found this unattractive and associated the shade with cholesterol, but perhaps because of our increasing habit of holidaying on the Continent and becoming more adventurous in our eating

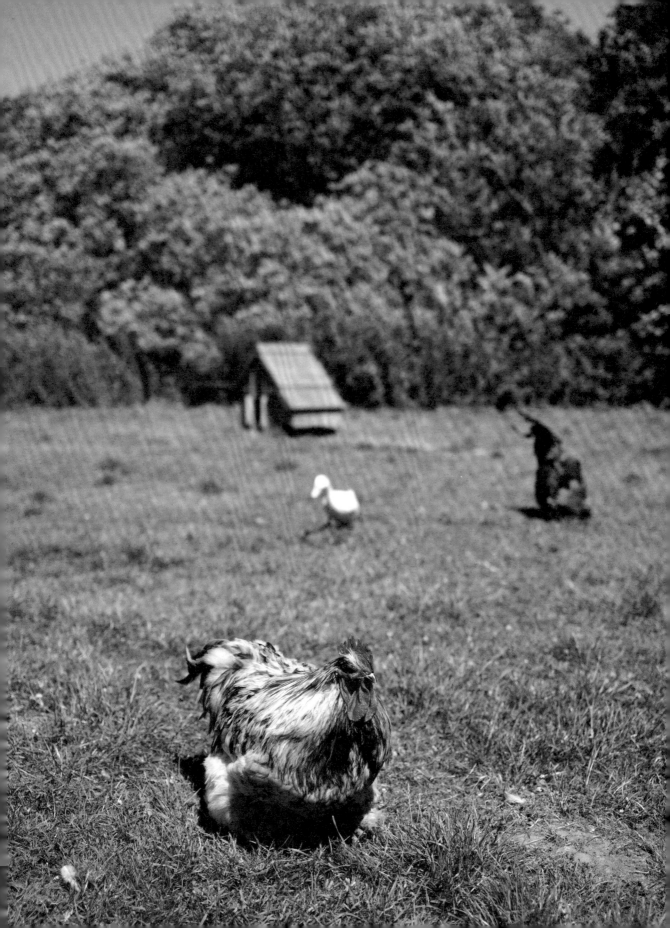

habits, 'corn-fed' chickens can now command a premium – and quite rightly so, as they are delicious.

Whatever you feed them on, chickens are marvellous converters of green and other waste matter into edible protein, be it eggs or meat. Then there is also, of course, the wonderful manure they produce. This is extremely acidic and so it will scorch plants when it is fresh, but it is also very high in nitrogen, so it is perfect for mixing with green garden waste as an activator to produce high-quality compost.

Benefits

Chickens are in many ways an ideal choice of livestock for the smallholder, whether for meat, eggs, or both. A chick from one of the big meat-producing breeds (a 'broiler') weighs about 50g, but immediately it begins to pile on the pounds. By the time it reaches six weeks old it will weigh about 3kg and be ready for slaughter.

Layers are generally lighter bodied and designed to pump every spare calorie into their eggs. Although a pullet won't start laying until she is four months old, she will then start to produce almost an egg a day for the rest of her life. Even if you have only two or three layers, most families will be pretty well self-sufficient in eggs – at least in summer (unless you provide artificial light to mimic at least 12 hours of daylight, production will tail off in the dark winter months).

Problems

The most obvious downside of chickens is that they will inevitably attract unwanted visitors in the form of rats and foxes. If you keep a cockerel to produce fertile eggs and create a healthy social structure among your flock, there can be noise problems and complaints from neighbours.

Breeds

Until recently, most chickens were dual-purpose breeds, designed to produce both eggs and meat. Over the last 50 years farmers have almost all switched to either an egg-laying or meat-producing specialist hybrid. The former can lay over 300 eggs a year, while the latter may reach killing weight in little more than a month.

There is still much to be said for the traditional varieties. Yes, a Light Sussex might grow slowly, but this can be turned to your advantage because the resulting flesh is denser and generally slightly darker than the commercial alternative. This not only adds to the flavour but also helps to distinguish the better-quality meat when it is on the shelf or on the plate. I am currently experimenting with small flocks of half-a-dozen breeds, collecting the eggs to hatch for sale as trios and for future stock. When the hens reach two years old they will be slaughtered to produce meat and stock for the restaurant.

BENEFITS OF NATURAL FORAGING

I witnessed an ingenious partial solution to the protein problem when I was filming in West Virginia. Joel Saladin had noticed his farm chickens naturally followed the cattle around, scratching at their pats. The lure was the beetle and fly larvae which lurked within. Inspired by this, Joel now puts his beef cattle in a field for a few weeks, then moves them out and his poultry in. The birds make a bee-line for the crusty pats, scratching vigorously at the surface to get at the grubs. Not only do Joel's birds get about 40 per cent of their protein needs in this way, but as they scratch away they scatter the mature manure across the ground, slashing his fertiliser bills.

The birds love the chance to indulge in such completely natural behaviour; as they scratch away they build up the leg muscles which will distinguish them from the mass-produced alternative. The obvious drawback here is that many customers would recoil at the thought of their meat coming from dung-scratching chickens , so you might need to market your birds as 'naturally foraged free-range chickens'!

One idea I am experimenting with at the farm is to plant small strips of fast-growing green plants which I can regularly harvest with a simple back-garden mower on the highest cut setting. This allows the crop to regenerate while the cut greens are tipped into the birds' run, where they will have great fun scratching and pecking through the pile.

You could do this with alfalfa, perpetual spinach or even leave it to weeds like chickweed and fat hen. Better still, you could plant it with a brassica such as kale or cabbage. In summer these greens will inevitably attract cabbage white butterflies, so when you give the leaves to your birds they can spend hours happily picking out the protein-rich caterpillars. This feed has two benefits: the insects will cut your expensive protein bills while the green material will boost their Omega 3 and 6 fat levels – again, something that can justify the birds' premium price tag.

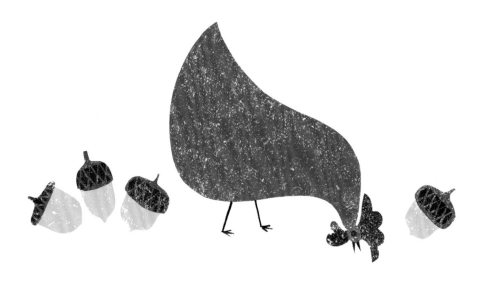

In the meantime, this breed also has the great benefit of looking magnificent – in marked contrast to the generally boring, white commercial hybrids. This will also help your marketing by giving you attractive images to put on your packaging and publicity. Better still, have the birds wandering around near your farm shop – preferably with one or two particularly docile examples in the car park who will happily peck and scratch around your visitors' feet.

Light Sussex: This is probably my favourite dual-purpose breed. There are various strains around, so be careful to select one of the biggest strains if keeping them for meat production is your main intention.

Rhode Island Reds: These birds are known mainly for their brown eggs, but the cockerels can produce a reasonable-sized table bird.

Marans: Another bird that is known mainly for its dark brown, lightly speckled eggs. Both the hens and the cockerels will also produce a decent table bird.

Indian game: Originally developed for cockfighting, these birds form the basis of most meat hybrids. You could produce your own by crossing a modern commercial meat game cockerel, then crossing this with another Indian game to produce a hardier, but slower-growing, big bird.

Barnvelders: These were originally developed in Holland and lay large dark brown eggs. They are very easy going and can become very tame.

Selling your produce

Whatever breed you opt for and however cleverly you market your meat, you are still implicitly competing against the mass-produced commercial roasting chickens which will always be sold at a significantly cheaper price than small suppliers could afford to sell at. This is largely due to buying food in bulk, housing indoors, stocking heavily and killing early, but it is also down to a hidden saving made at the abattoir: big producers deliver tens of thousands of birds to the highly mechanised production lines every day. As a result, it costs just a few pence to transform a hen into a potential roasting joint.

How are you going to kill, pluck, gut and truss your bird? You can do it by hand in the traditional manner, of course, but this takes time. However skilled you might become, you are unlikely to be able to prepare more than a couple of birds per hour – not least because traditional breeds have more feathers and fluff than hybrids.

One solution is to work out a deal with a commercial neighbour or even to talk directly to the abattoir. If you are lucky they will tack your crate of birds on at the end of the day, but whatever you do, don't embark on producing meat-producing birds until you have worked out a solution to this most basic of problems.

The main drawback with chickens, from a commercial point of view, is their very popularity. As a nation on average we each eat 180 eggs and 23kg of chicken

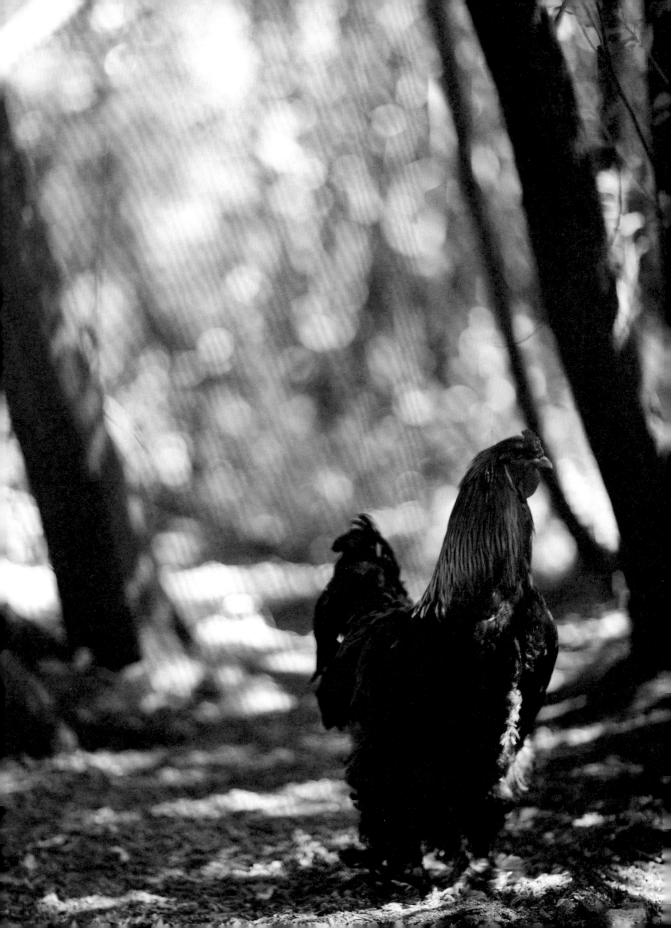

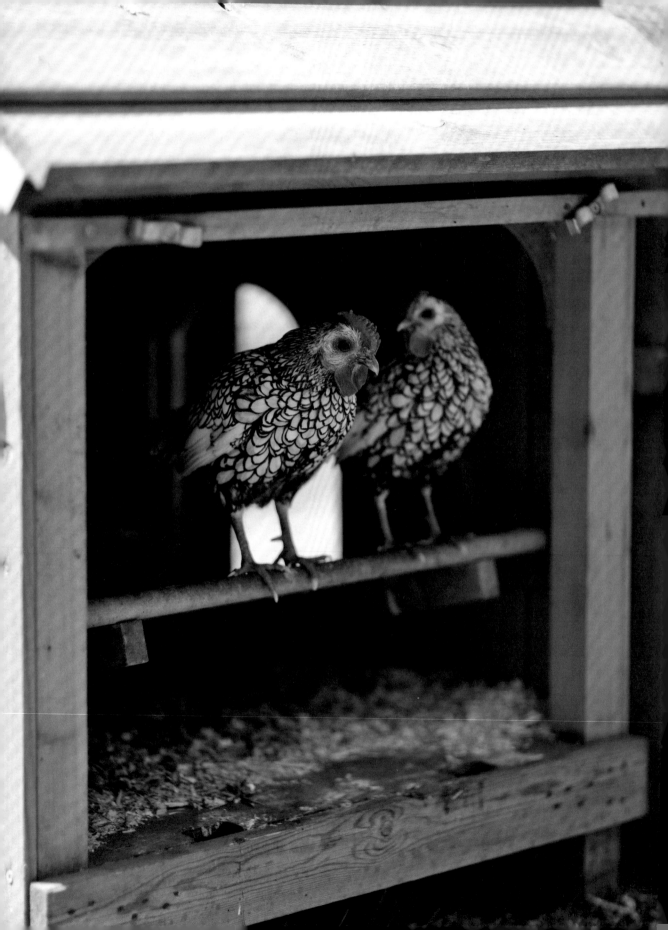

every year, but until the 1950s chicken was a luxury, found only at the tables of the rich. Up until then older birds – hens – that had finished their egg-laying lives might often appear on butchers' slabs as 'boiling fowl', but the only young, tender birds to be killed were the surplus cockerels or 'capons', which were redundant because they would obviously never produce eggs. Even so, in the days before modern fast-growing hybrids, these birds took several months to become fully grown, which meant their meat was expensive.

After the privations of the Second World War, followed by the growing prosperity of the 1950s and 1960s, enterprising businessmen looked hard at the way we produced all our meat and realised that by revolutionising poultry keeping there was a source of cheap, profitable protein. Instead of keeping relatively small free-range flocks of dual-purpose (egg and meat) breeds, output could be hugely increased by breeding fast-growing hybrids, increasing numbers and crowding them indoors to reduce expensive food being burnt off as the birds exercised and kept warm. It also greatly reduced problems from predators. These businessmen also looked at the chickens' food, bumping up the protein content with either fish or soya meal, and developed specialised abattoirs which could stun, bleed, pluck and gut thousands of chickens an hour for just a few pence each.

The results have been – on one level at least – spectacularly successful. While older breeds struggle to reach killing weight before they are four or five months old, modern hybrids like the Ross Cobb can weigh as much as 4–5kg in just 42 days (in fact, in many birds the flesh grows so fast that the bone structure can't keep up and their hips give way). As a result, virtually all the oven-ready chickens you see on your supermarket shelf have been killed at just six weeks. This produces very pale soft flesh with comparatively little flavour – but that, it seems, is what we as a nation have come to expect in our meat. In contrast the French delay slaughter until 84 days and routinely feed their birds on more expensive maize – which explains why even their commercial fowl are more expensive but have more texture and flavour.

Now, this history lesson is important because it explains why the smallholder will never be able to compete with the big boys on price when it comes to meat production. Unless you want to go down the factory farming route, you will struggle to produce any oven-ready bird for less than two or three times the price of the supermarket roaster.

However, this doesn't rule out keeping hens for saleable meat. Although small-scale poultry-keepers will always produce expensive birds, thanks to recent high-profile campaigns by celebrity chefs, food writers and animal rights activists there is a growing market for high-quality meat from happy animals. The problem is that because this meat will cost several times as much as a conventional bird, you need to think imaginatively about how you would market your product range.

How to add value to your produce

Let's assume you have solved the plucking and gutting problem; the next issue is how to convince your customers to pay for the privilege of eating your product. The smallholder will never be able to compete on price. You will struggle to produce any oven-ready bird for less than three times the price of the supermarket roaster.

So, if you are selling your birds as roasters, make sure they are as attractively packaged as possible. For example, put in a big bunch of an appropriate herb such as lemon thyme or tarragon and a package of assorted organic vegetables to serve alongside the finished roast. This way as the customer opens their purchase on Sunday morning, they are greeted with a wonderful waft of fresh herbs, garlic and leek – all of which goes to reinforce their impression of having acquired not just a meal, but a real treat.

It's also worth taking a leaf from the supermarkets' books. They may be able to sell an oven-ready bird for £3, but you will notice their cold shelves have even more packs of skinned breasts, thighs, drumsticks and wings. If you tot up the price of the individual cuts versus the whole bird, you will see there's a very significant mark-up. Even if you allow for the discarded bones, I reckon jointing a chicken can double its retail price – and the silly thing is the process couldn't be easier! It takes half-a-dozen cuts of the knife to transform a whole bird into the six simplest joints. Anyone can do it, but it seems most modern consumers are quite happy to pay you a lot of money to save them the trouble. Assuming you have identified an abattoir willing to pluck and gut your birds you could ask them to cut them up, but it is very easy to do it yourself. You will need, however, to have an approved cutting room.

Portioning your birds also allows you to turn the cheapest cuts into upmarket products. Wings, for example, are normally virtually thrown away. This is a tragedy because, as with all animals, the fatty flesh next to the bone is actually the sweetest meat. In summer supermarkets sometimes marinate these in Indian or Chinese-style flavourings, but you could do much better by creating your own recipes using home-grown herbs, fruit or honey. The other 'brown meat' cuts from the legs may be worth more, but this can also be increased in value – perhaps by dicing, marinating in a different range of flavourings, and then skewering to make kebabs. You could then put both along with some home-grown organic vegetables in a 'barbecue box'.

One step further is to tap into the modern taste for ready meals. Customers may be increasingly prepared to pay for quality, but not everyone has the skill, time or desire to cook from scratch. Your chicken could become a delicious home-baked pie, casserole or curry – sold fresh, frozen or even delivered to the door. The list is endless, but as so often it can be a good idea to wander down the aisles

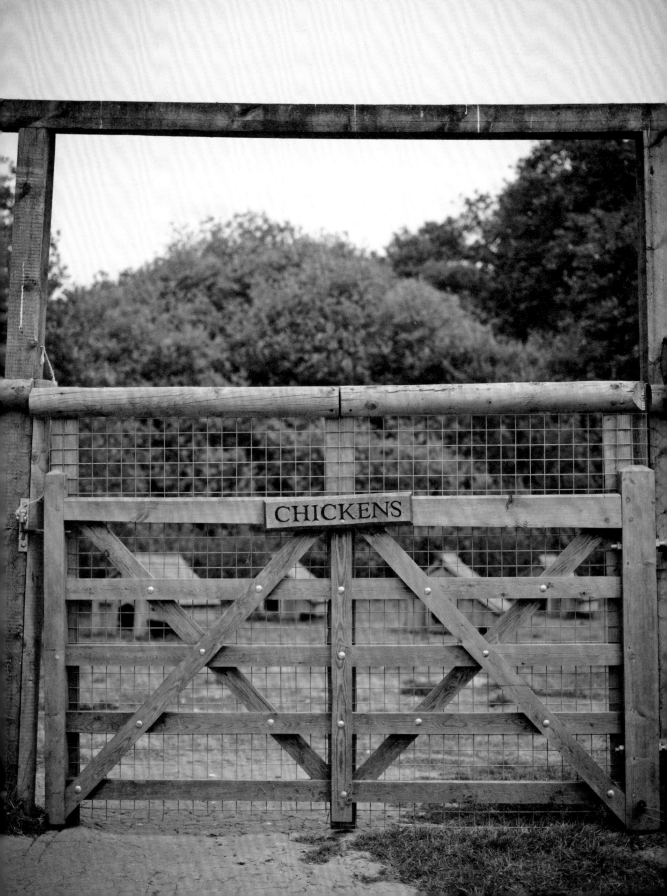

of local food shops – both supermarket and specialist – to get an idea of what is already selling well. Using this as a pointer you could then devise your own products, perhaps basing these on a favourite family dish cooked by a grandmother, or maybe turning to traditional local recipes researched from old cookery books.

Another very simple process is to cook the meat by smoking it. This slowly steams the bird in a smokey atmosphere to create a wonderfully moist picnic or salad ingredient. You can vary the product by altering the wood chips or sawdust you are using – or throw a handful of herbs onto the fire. Or you could go one stage further and mix the flaked flesh with homemade mayonnaise, semi-dried tomatoes and nuts to create an interesting variation on the classic coronation chicken.

The other aspect to consider is that while you might be doubling your chicken's value by breaking it down into its component parts, you are also creating a potentially valuable waste product. Most of your customers would probably throw the skin and bones into the bin, but if you roast these briefly in a hot oven to brown them, then simmer them in hot water with onion, leek, carrot and some bay leaves you will make a fantastic richly coloured stock.

This is what we aim to do with our two-year-old hens after they've finished their second laying season. Our stock will go into the restaurant, but you could sell this straight (either fresh or frozen) as something which is infinitely superior to dried cubes of instant stock. Better still, combine it with home-grown vegetables to create soups (chicken and sweetcorn, leek and potato, or tomato and basil spring to mind). Or think of it as a component in the 'ingredient' equivalent of a veggie box – packaged up with a few fresh vegetables, local hard cheese and short-grain rice as a 'risotto kit'.

The possibilities are endless, but the important point is that every time you add something to your product you can bump up its selling price. The more little elements and flourishes you can factor in, the more you are able to justify charging a sensible price to cover the huge input of time and effort that will almost inevitably go into your finished product.

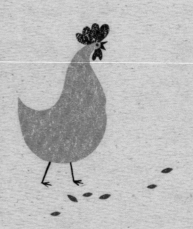

THE CRAFT OF SMOKING FOOD

Smoking is a delicious and simple way to preserve food. There are two main forms – cold and hot – but both are perfect ways to prepare a huge range of produce.

Although today the process is mainly used as flavouring, it was originally developed as a way to preserve food in the days before refrigeration. The smoke contains anti-bacterial agents, but the preservative qualities stem mainly from dehydration. Products typically lose about 30 per cent of their weight (which explains one reason for the increase in value). Obviously much of this drying comes as the food hangs in the smoke column, but it usually begins with light salting beforehand. This comes either by being rubbed with dry salt or by soaking in brine (this is often given additional flavourings such as molasses, herbs or alcohol).

The produce then hangs in a smoke column for several hours, or even days, depending on its size and shape and the qualities you are aiming to achieve. Scallops or mussels, for example, might need just a few minutes, cheese could require a couple of hours, while oils or a ham could hang for several days.

Smoking is a craft. You can read specialist books on the subject (better still, visit a smokery and ask lots of questions), but in the end the only way to perfect the process is by trial and error, so a good tip is to start with cheap materials. Trout is ideal because it is cheap and delicious (both cold- and hot-smoked, thus temperature mistakes are not critical). Once you can consistently get good results, move onto pork bellies, poultry or vegetables – again, comparatively cheap ingredients which mean your inevitable mistakes will not prove costly. Finally, try smoking cheese or hams to produce premium ingredients.

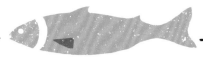

✔ HOT SMOKING

Sometimes called 'cook' smoking, this is the easier process. Until recently it has been more popular on the Continent and in the United States than in Britain (although smoked mackerel and kippers are notable exceptions). As the name suggests, it uses warm smoke (generally 65–93°C). The heat changes the texture of the raw material to produce something which is clearly cooked. The process produces lots of flavour, but it is only a mild preservative.

✔ COLD SMOKING

As its name suggests, this uses cooler fumes (39–43°C). It is generally the slower process, typically taking at least 12 hours (many more for a big ham) and it creates longer-lasting products (typically extending the shelf-life three- or four-fold). When done well it produces superior results, but not surprisingly it requires more care and skill. This is the way conventional smoked salmon is created, but it is also ideal for products you want to flavour without actually cooking. For example salami, ham and cheese can respond well.

DIY SMOKEHOUSE

It is easy to make a smoker; this is basically a simple chamber where the produce is bathed in woodsmoke. This can be any size or shape, but remember that if you intend to cold smoke even smouldering sawdust is burning at several hundred degrees, so keeping the temperature down is the biggest problem. As a result, a tall chamber will allow you to suspend your produce at a range of heights (with, obviously, the coolest at the top). Another way to lower the temperature is to have the fire chamber a few yards away and to feed in the smoke through a metal pipe. This not only makes the smoke cooler, but it reduces the smell and risk of a costly fire. The chamber should have several vents at both bottom and top to allow you to control the temperature and airflow, while inside it needs a variety of racks and hangers to allow you to process a range of produce.

This smokehouse can also be used to hot smoke by moving the fire inside the chamber, but if you are only interested in hot-smoking, then making a smoker is even simpler: a metal dustbin with hooks bolted to the underside of the lid will work fine.

Generating the smoke can be a little more difficult than you might think. Shavings and whole sticks are easiest to keep alight, but require much more attention, not least because they often flare to produce excess heat. This not only cooks the food, but the hotter the fire, the less smoke it generates. As a result smouldering sawdust is a safer option, although it can often go out. One easy solution is to put the sawdust in an old frying pan on an electric ring in the bottom of the chamber. When it begins to smoke, turn the heat and vents down low.

The safest bet of all is to buy a ready-made, semi-professional model. The Bradley smoker, for example, is an electric kiln generating smoke from blocks of compressed sawdust (see www.bradleysmoker.co.uk), but you can also buy much cheaper portable versions from fishing and camping shops. These are often little more than large tins containing a grill and they can only hot smoke.

✓ WHAT FUEL?

The wood used is critical to the final product. In Britain oak is the most popular timber, giving the produce a distinctive fuller flavour. Alternatively, fruit trees such as apple or cherry will impart a sweeter quality. In America, hickory and mesquite are more popular. Whatever wood is used, it must be a hardwood; conifers have far too much resin which will taint the produce with the scent and taste of creosote. For the same reason, even hardwood should be fairly dry to reduce the tar content.

You can buy a range of special smoke briquettes on the internet or from many outdoor shops, but this can work out to be quite expensive. An easy alternative is to ask a joiner or wood turner for their sawdust and shavings. Most will be only too pleased to get rid of their waste and can even supply you with a range of unusual timbers.

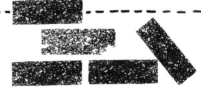

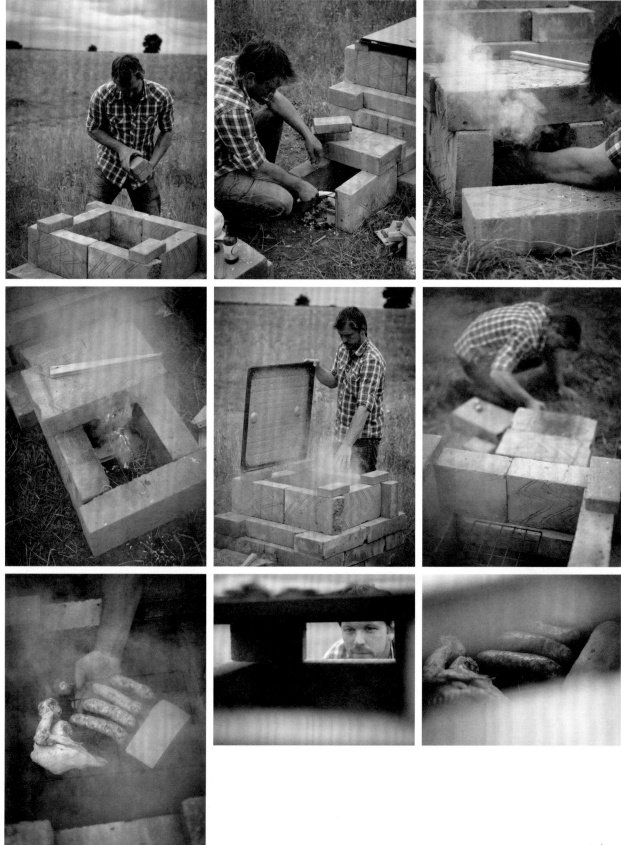

CASE STUDY »

CASE STUDY

Michael Leviseur began EXPERIMENTING with Smoking Food in the 1980s, But decided to turn it into a BUSINESS in the 1990s when he and his Wife Debbie Moved to a RAMBLing farmhouse in Clunbury, South SHROPSHIRE.

It was a brave move, because not only is the trade dominated by big commercial players, but there are dozens of small smokeries scattered across the country, all of which turn out a bewildering range of products.

This meant that from the start the Leviseurs needed to find a marketing angle to make their business stand out from the crowd. The first step was the methodology. Most smokeries use commercial kilns – huge ovens with fans to circulate the smoke around the produce. In contrast Michael looked to the past, when farmers and fishermen would simply hang their produce in the chimney where it was slowly bathed in the rising smoke, sometimes for several days.

So Michael constructed his own version of this smoking chimney, building simple wooden chambers where the wood (which always comes from air-dried timber from naturally fallen local oaks) smoulders at the bottom. This requires great skill because outside temperature and humidity play an important role in determining the density of the smoke and how long the process will take.

As a result Michael has to be constantly on hand to manually adjust the air vents on each chamber to control the smoking speed. He says that even after 20 years he is still learning the art: which explains why, to this day, he is Britain's only commercial chimney smoker. Having put in all this effort to

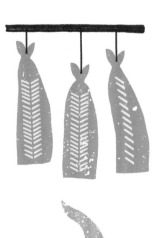

devise a unique craft, it was then only natural to register with the Soil Association.

From the start the couple knew it was vital to establish a premium reputation if the business was to succeed. Clearly the quality of the ingredients is vital and their most important line, smoked salmon, is based on organically farmed fish reared right out at sea on the east coast of Lewis. 'It's more expensive, but much purer than other farmed salmon, which comes from sheltered sea lochs where there is less ebb and flow of water,' he explains.

Once harvested, the fish is immediately freighted overnight to south Shropshire where it is layered with Maldon salt to lightly dry cure. The excess salt is then rinsed off and the fish is air-dried before being smoked. This is important because almost all rival products are brine-cured and put into the smoke still damp. By contrast, the Leviseurs' salmon is much paler and drier because there are no chemicals or colourings; this also gives it a more subtle flavour. The hard work has clearly been worth it because The Smokeyard has won a stream of awards every year, consistently beating the major supermarkets – a fact which gives Michael particular satisfaction.

Their product range is much greater than just their take on smoked salmon. They also produce a hot-smoked version, not to mention smoked versions of chicken breast, Parmesan, sea salt and even olive oil. With this range of unusual organic ingredients, it's not surprising that this Marches' business should catch the attention of top chefs, with Rick Stein, Gordon Ramsay, Nigella Lawson and Jamie Oliver among the list of celebrity customers.

'Smoked salmon has always been the core business,' explains Debbie. 'But we also do a lot of smoking to order for local chefs. They usually come to us with an idea for, say, smoked fillet of venison and if it sounds interesting we try to oblige.' Thus one restaurant has a weekly order of smoked milk, while their butter is popular as an ingredient in unusual hollandaise and béchamel sauces. Debbie says that while this is only a minor part of their business financially, these bepoke products are fun and interesting.

More importantly, however, it makes for brilliant marketing: 'When one chef puts something quirky on the menu it attracts the attention of other chefs – better still, it is the quirky unusual stuff which gets written about in the press.'

'The secret to success is to have a total belief in your product,' grins Michael. 'If you're not convinced your salmon is the best, how on earth are you going to sell it to a hesitating customer on a cold market stall in February?'

Ducks

Almost all domesticated ducks are descended from the mallard – the only exception being the Muscovy, which traces its roots to a South American species. Most domesticated duck breeds are considerably larger and more prolific than their wild forebears. A mallard drake weighs about 1kg while the duck generally lays a clutch of about 12 eggs. In contrast a fully grown Aylesbury duckling can weigh 6kg and a Khaki Campbell can lay 300 eggs a year.

Benefits

The right breed of duck is as prolific as any hen, laying large rich eggs which are often covered with a gorgeous blue-green shell. If you want meat, then they are quick-growing (ducklings are ready for the table at eight weeks) and they have modest space requirements – although they certainly need to be housed at night. Ducks are also great fun – waddling and quacking contentedly around the garden and, better still, they seem to love slugs and snails (unlike chickens, which turn their beaks up at slimy gastropods).

Problems

If chickens tend to attract pests and predators, this is even more so with ducks. Foxes will jump six-foot fences to get at them, while rats will readily kill the ducklings with a bite to the back of the head. Ducks also have a significant amount of feathers – not to mention a thick underlayer of fluffy down. In former times these were used to stuff pillows and quilts, but doing this is difficult if you have many birds. Today most birds destined for market are 'wet-plucked' by being immersed briefly in scalding water before the feathers are mechanically ripped from the skin. This results in a soggy mix of feather and down which includes a fair amount of blood and fat. Of course, you can hand-pluck the feathers and down, but the thickness of the layers means this is extremely time-consuming. The feathers do contain plenty of nitrogen, however, so they are great as a compost additive.

Breeds

There are plenty of duck breeds to choose from. Most are big, and so even the egg-laying strains are dual-purpose to some extent. The best breed is therefore likely to be the one you find most attractive.

Aylesbury: This is one of the biggest ducks (averaging about 5kg) and is

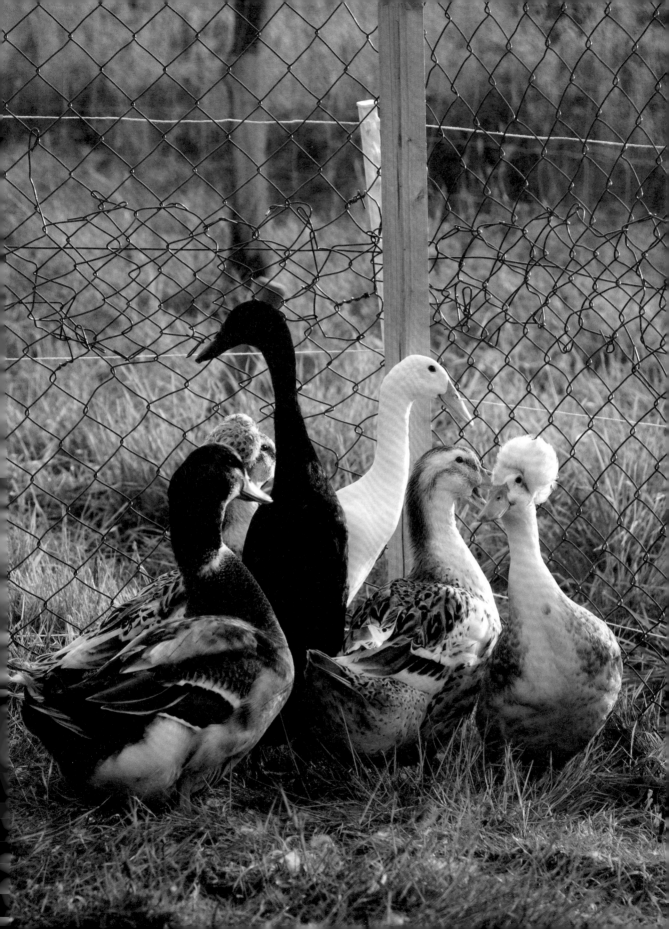

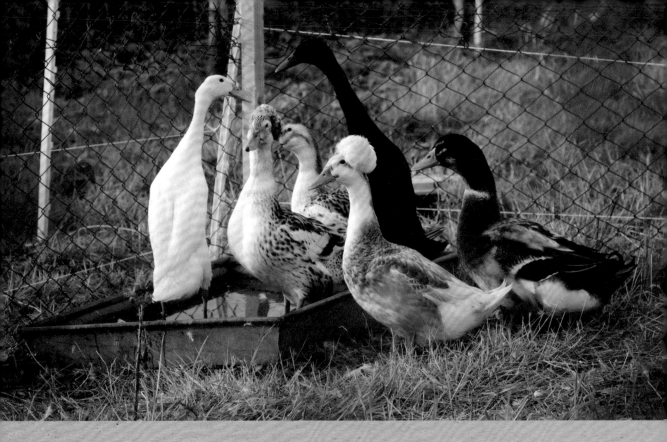

Britain's most popular meat breed. As with all large ducks and geese, fertility can be a problem. This can be overcome by crossing a smaller, more agile drake with large ducks and by providing a moderately deep pool in which to mate.

Indian runner: An unusually upright breed (immortalised in the film *Babe*), it is very active and light bodied so it is usually kept for laying rather than for its carcass.

Khaki Campbell: A prolific layer (averaging 300 eggs a year), this is the result of crosses between mallard, Rouen and runner ducks. It is also a relatively large bird and therefore dual purpose.

Muscovy: Despite its name, this is a domesticated South American species often regarded as a small goose rather than duck. Its meat is comparatively

gamey and dark, but is also very large (6kg for ducks and 8kg for drakes). It is particularly popular in France, where it is known as the Barbary. Foie gras producers often cross it with Rouens to reduce the gaminess of the flesh while maintaining the size.

Pekin (Long Island): The most popular American meat breed traces its roots to domesticated Chinese mallards. It typically grows to about 4–5kg.

Silver Appleyard: This beautiful breed was developed during the 1940s. Its developer, Reginald Appleyard, said his aim was to make 'a beautiful breed of duck, with a combination of size, beauty and lots of big white eggs'. These qualities and their docile nature make them ideal for back-garden production.

Selling your produce

If you are thinking of rearing ducks as a commercial enterprise, you need to decide whether your prime aim is to sell the eggs or meat – each process has its own pros and cons. That said, bear in mind that many breeds are dual purpose, so even if your main aim is to produce eggs, if you are hatching future laying stock from fertile eggs, one in two eggs is going to produce a drake – and he is never going to produce an egg.

Ducks grow almost as fast as chickens, and if they are being reared for meat they will be ready at eight weeks old. Commercial birds are kept in huge indoor flocks, so there is a clear opening for naturally reared, outdoor, free-range birds. These will have more muscle and therefore taste better than the intensively reared equivalent.

Unfortunately, while a duck may be worth two or three times as much as a chicken, be warned that most supermarkets now stock oven-ready birds at a price you cannot hope to match. In Britain most ducks are intended for roasting whole, but in many parts of Europe – most notably France's Languedoc – farmers add value by turning each bird into a range of products. The breast fillets make prime cuts for searing on a griddle or under a grill, while the legs are potted in their own fat as 'confit' or mixed with beans, tomatoes and sausages to make cassoulet. Finally, the livers are often turned into a rich pâté – or the birds are force fed grain for the last fortnight of life to produce the melting succulent and rich foie gras (literally, 'fat liver').

Traditionally this force feeding is done by putting a funnel in the bird's beak and literally forcing pre-soaked maize down its throat two or three times a day (this is called 'gavage'). This process is generally regarded as cruel and is banned in many countries, although some American farmers have developed 'cruelty-free' fattening techniques which encourage the birds to gorge themselves at the time when their wild ancestors would be migrating (because then they are naturally inclined to pile on the calories and build up fat reserves). Whether this actually produces a liver to match the quality of the force-fed duck is debatable, but it is legal and certainly more ethically acceptable to many consumers.

Eggs are a much less questionable duck product. Some breeds, such as Khaki Campbells, are prolific layers. Ducks' eggs are a little larger and richer than hens' eggs and, being less widely available, they are worth about twice as much, although finding a steady market can be difficult.

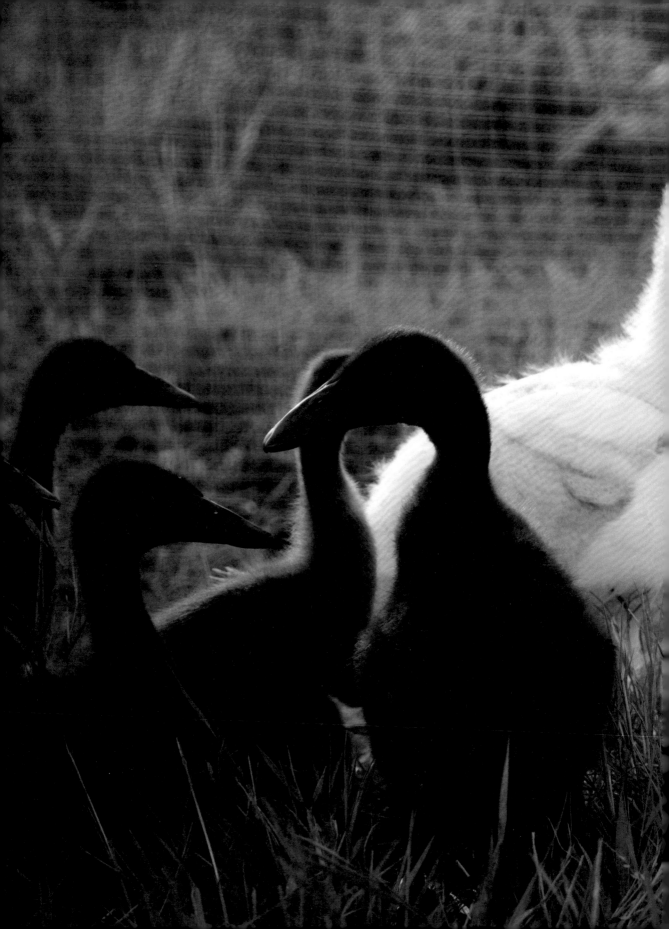

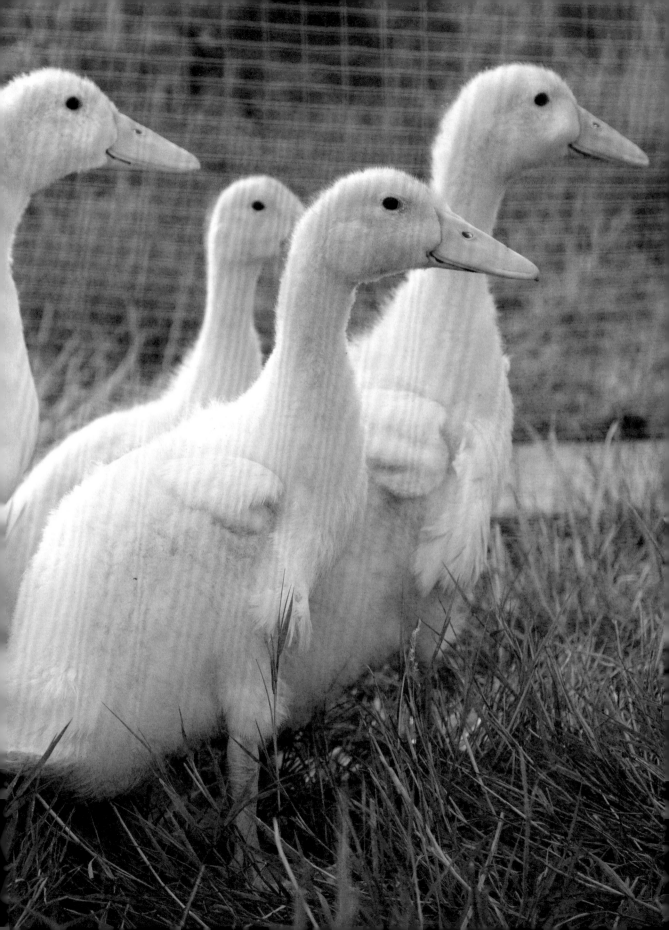

Geese

Most European domesticated geese are descended from the wild greylag goose, while Asian breeds come from the swan goose. However, as with ducks, they are often much larger than their ancestors, with the biggest unable to fly (although, as I know from bitter experience, they can take off and plane downhill in a high wind).

Benefits

You might think geese are just bigger versions of ducks, but this isn't so. Ducks are omnivores that need protein if they are to put on weight or produce eggs, which means that realistically you need to buy in food for them. Geese, on the other hand, are largely vegetarian and are happy to nibble their way across your lawn or field, only needing supplementary feeding with maize or corn in the last two or three weeks of their lives in early winter. These birds are also hardy, and once they have grown their feathers they need no protection from the elements – although they do need to be locked away at night to protect them from foxes. They do swim, obviously, but they don't necessarily require water (their wild ancestors spend most of the day grazing on land). They do love dabbling in water, though, and the bigger breeds can only mate with its help, so if you want fertile eggs from, say, an Emden or Toulouse, you will need to provide a pond.

Problems

As so often is the case, many of their advantages have a negative side. Geese are very seasonal birds in that, unlike chickens and ducks, an adult goose lays a limited number of eggs during a comparatively short spring window, not least because while their diet may make them a great way of turning grass into protein, it's a slow process. A chicken can be oven-ready at six weeks, but a goose takes closer to six months. This is because their digestive systems are very inefficient, so while each one may eat kilos of grass every day, almost all reappears within a few hours as green slimy tubes that soon cover the ground around them. As a result, while you can see their front end as a wonderful walking mower, their back ends will be churning out manure all over your cherished lawn for the whole of the late spring, summer and early autumn, ruling them out for most proud gardeners.

Geese are very territorial creatures, and while they can make good security guards (remember the geese warning the Romans of the Goth attack on the Capitol?), your neighbours might not appreciate their clamours of outrage every time you have a caller.

If you are hoping to turn your geese into profit, their value could be an issue. Foxes just adore geese, particularly when the first frosts of the winter add an edge to their appetites, and at £50 for an oven-ready Christmas bird, any loss will really sting. Worse still, unlike chickens or ducks, it also means you have to guard against light-fingered humans.

Breeds

Geese are derived from several wild species, so their domesticated descendants can vary greatly in size and temperament. Thus it is important to start with a breed that fits your purpose and it's well worth buying good stock.

Chinese: A smaller breed which lays a lot of eggs (maybe 70–80 each spring). It is noisy, so makes a good burglar alarm, but it produces a small carcass.

Toulouse: One of the biggest breeds, weighing up to 9kg, as its name suggests this comes originally from south-west France where it produces the finest foie gras livers.

Emden: Originating in Germany, this large white bird is the principal commercial breed, growing quickly to about 9–14kg.

Selling your produce

Until the late nineteenth century, goose was the roast of choice for the festive season. For much of the last century its place was supplanted by the faster-growing, bigger-breasted turkey, but more recently goose has recovered in popularity. Fortunately for the small producer, the fact that goose fattens so slowly means it has never lent itself to mass production. As a result it rarely appears on supermarket shelves and instead consumers generally have to turn to traditional butchers or upmarket mail-order suppliers to get hold of a bird. This means it is rightly regarded as a luxury product and has a high price tag to match. At the time of writing, by weight an oven-ready goose is worth about five times as much as a duck.

Alternatively, you can take a leaf from that great geese-producing region, the Languedoc, where the birds are processed into a range of high-value products such as confit, cassoulet and foie gras. Foie gras is an alternative product (most gourmets rate fattened goose livers as the best, although these only account for 4 per cent of French foie gras production), but, as with ducks, force-feeding leads to serious legal and ethical issues.

Goose feathers and down are more highly rated than those of ducks, and these could possibly be an earner – although the same problems with how to produce clean dry feathers in quantity crop up. Even a skilled plucker can spend the best part of an hour preparing a goose, so yet again most birds are usually either wet-plucked mechanically or waxed.

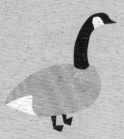

Turkeys

These large-breasted birds are the domesticated descendants of an American game bird, so they were unknown in Europe until the seventeenth century. At this time they began to be reared in East Anglia and driven to market, but they remained a luxury food until after the Second World War (the Cratchit family was going to make do with goose until the repentant Scrooge gave them a turkey in *A Christmas Carol*). In the 1950s, however, their intensive-farming potential was spotted and they rapidly became first the nation's favourite Christmas dinner, then one of the cheapest staple meats (particularly when frozen or processed to make burgers and breadcrumbed or battered shapes).

Benefits

Most turkey breeds are quick-growing, with a 24-week stag weighing up to 16kg and a hen 10kg. Their size means they are also great to portion into smaller joints. Their meat is also very healthy, low in fat and cholesterol, so is much loved by the health-conscious, and although they are indelibly associated with Christmas turkey is good to eat at any time of year. The birds are relatively hardy and will find much of their own food if allowed to wander across grass – and the stags can be particularly striking once they develop their wattles and tail fans.

Problems

Turkeys can be noisy. Personally I think their chattering rattles are charming, but this can lead to problems with neighbours. Also, some lighter traditional breeds are surprisingly good fliers, taking off in the evening to perch on branches. In theory this lifts them out of the way of predators, but in practice they are much safer locked away at night.

Breeds

There are fewer turkey breeds than there are chickens or ducks, but there is still a good choice. Some of the bigger breeds have also been developed to have fewer feathers. This may be useful if you intend plucking them yourself, but they will not be as hardy as some of their traditional counterparts.

Bronze: A beautifully feathered bird, hence the name bronze, this is a slow-growing strain which as a result produces great-tasting meat.

Broad-breasted white: This is your archetypal commercial strain. It's favoured by the poultry industry because any pin feathers that remain after plucking are less visible against its pale skin.

Norfolk black: Probably Britain's most popular traditional breed, this still grows to a large size and many consumers associate the remaining dark pin feathers with quality and being free range.

Bourbon red: Named after Bourbon County in Kentucky, this is a smaller, traditional breed with striking rusty plumage. Stags can weigh up to 16kg, but are generally slaughtered at about half this weight.

Selling your produce

If you are thinking about rearing turkeys for sale, be aware that since the 1950s turkeys have been farmed intensively by big producers, which has driven the price down and given the birds a reputation for poor quality. Worse, the effort involved in producing huge birds with ever-bigger breasts means that some are unable to breed naturally while others suffer from hip problems because their soft growing bones cannot cope with the weight of their bodies. This has further lowered consumer attitudes towards the meat.

Big oven-ready birds have a limited seasonal market, so portioning and adding value is a good way to spread sales throughout the year. The history of processed turkey products is not a happy one (remember Jamie Oliver's campaign against the turkey twizzler?), but in fact the relatively delicate meat can be turned into a range of interesting products. For example it smokes well to make a delicate buffet meat, while the great size of the bird makes it perfect for boning and stuffing with a range of other meats – such as boned chicken, duck, pheasant or quail. After roasting, this can be sliced to make a premium version of the Elizabethan delicacy of a swan stuffed with a peacock, goose, capon, pheasant and partridge. If you are pre-cooking turkey for sale, however, remember that because the flesh is low on fat, it can dry out quickly.

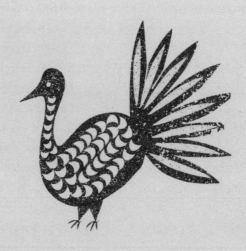

CASE STUDY »

CASE STUDY KellyBronze Turkeys

The KELLY family have been rearing TURKEYS since 1971, and over the years they have built up a THRIVING Business that has become a RECOGNISED brand LEADER well beyond their Native ESSEX.

However, it hasn't always been plain sailing, according to Paul, the second generation to run the KellyBronze company, but he says he still gets as much satisfaction from his turkeys as he did when he started off in the business.

The company began in 1971 when Paul's father, Derek, began to import breeding stock from Oregon, although this was really a sideline: 'We fed and reared the turkeys, while Dad did consultancy work in Europe,' explains Paul. All the same, competition from big producers and tight margins meant that by the early 1980s the business was almost going under.

The problem was that in those days the market was split between big growers who supplied the supermarkets with frozen birds and traditional butchers who sold fresh turkeys produced on small family-run farms. Prices could – and did – fluctuate wildly depending on the numbers produced each year, and the vagaries of the market meant it was easy for a small producer to lose a lot of money.

The Kellys decided the solution was to concentrate on quality. This meant going back to the traditional slow-growing bronze turkey and rearing them in free-range conditions. So, while big producers slaughter their white-feathered birds at 12 weeks, a Kelly turkey takes six months to mature. This results in a full-flavoured meat with a dense texture. 'We were only just in time – the strain had almost died out,' says Paul. 'We bought the last 350 bronze turkeys we could find and crossed them all to try to get the broadest genetic base to avoid in-breeding.'

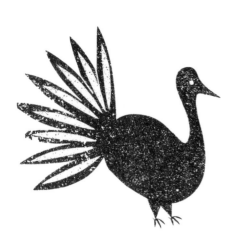

The quality of the meat is ensured further by dry plucking the carcasses and then hanging these for a couple of weeks to enhance the taste and texture. The problem was that while this produced a clearly superior product, it was sometimes difficult to get the message across. 'All these little farms supplying local butchers meant it was a very fragmented market,' explains Paul. 'It was difficult to tell the public that this was a premium product.'

To complicate matters further, salmonella scares over poultry saw the introduction of a raft of new health and hygiene regulations in the mid-80s: 'It meant everyone had to up their game,' says Paul. 'This put a lot of pressure on all turkey farmers and it was certainly a nightmare for us – we had no money and by the end of 1986 I remember thinking, "We're not going to make this."'

Fortunately, the Kellys' timing was just right. 'It was the beginning of the foodie revolution and this was a good-news story about a traditional breed,' explains Paul. The business attracted just enough media interest to bring in the orders. The real breakthrough came when Delia Smith interviewed the family in 1990. More importantly, she featured their birds in her Christmas book. 'That was when everything took off,' says Paul. 'It gave us momentum, we borrowed money and pumped everything into the business.'

More recently they have begun training others to rear birds to their own exacting standards. Becoming a KellyBronze farmer offers valuable savings for the farmer. 'They rear the birds free-range within sight of a reasonably busy road, then we process, pluck and hang them before returning them to sell direct to the public,' says Paul. 'This means we get the wholesale margin while the KellyBronze farmer gets the retail margin.'

After years of experience the Kellys have developed a tried-and-tested formula to make turkeys profitable for the smallholder. This means living within 15 minutes of at least 20,000 people, having at least two acres of free range, an attractive, tidy farm with barns capable of housing the birds at night and in bad weather, plus a readiness to rear the birds to Kelly specifications.

One might have thought that the seasonal nature of the business would be a problem, but Paul believes it is actually a huge advantage. 'The positive aspect for the small producer is that they know exactly when their sales are coming, so everyone can muck in together for a short period,' he says. 'You do very long days for a few weeks in the run-up to Christmas, but then it's all over.' Another advantage is that people will pay a decent price for a premium product in the festive season.

Certainly the Kellys' business has gone from strength to strength over the past 15 years or so, and is now bringing in an annual turnover of £7.5 million, including its franchises. 'I love my birds and the 40-odd years I've spent with them,' says Paul. 'There's a tremendous satisfaction in knowing they are the best turkeys you can buy.'

Quails

These small migratory game birds are popular in Mediterranean cookery and their eggs have long been considered a delicacy. Although the quail that appear on menus in the Middle East and Southern Europe are generally shot as they migrate to and from their African wintering grounds, they have been domesticated since Roman times. A few hundred migrate here every summer, but the eggs that appear in delicatessens and good butchers are all domesticated versions of the Japanese variety. The carcasses occasionally appear on cold shelves (on the Continent they are more valued for their carcasses which are often crunched up whole: bones and all), but the principal demand here is for their beautiful mottled eggs which are hard-boiled to make canapés.

Benefits

If poultry generally has modest space requirements, then quail are super compact and are prolific layers. It is perfectly possible to keep several dozen in a small ark which can be moved around even the tiniest garden to allow them to hunt for insects amongst the grass. An alternative is to put them in wall-mounted hutches like the wire-fronted shelves old-fashioned pet shops used for displaying canaries – although this is too close to battery farming for my liking.

That said, stemming originally from warmer climes, quails are delicate and benefit from being moved indoors at night. It is also worth pointing out that as game birds they need a higher-protein diet than chickens or ducks, particularly in winter: pheasant rearing crumbs are the best solution.

It's also worth saying that while you will need the prolific Japanese Corturnix variety if you want to produce eggs for sale, several other species have also been domesticated. The American bobwhite and Californian varieties are very pretty and make colourful additions, in particular in gardens where space is at a premium.

Problems

As I've already said, these are fairly delicate birds and they need protection from frost and wet, so they can't live outside all year round. As a small bird they are also vulnerable to a particularly wide range of predators. As well as the usual foxes and rats, stoats, weasels, sparrowhawks and domestic cats are a serious threat, so they will always need to be kept protected at all times and from every direction.

Although they readily lay fertile eggs, hatching these to keep up a steady supply of eggs in future can be tricky. The chicks are tiny when they emerge from the egg and very vulnerable to chilling. The biggest risk is damp, so they are best kept indoors in a fish tank under a heat lamp. Their pelvises are also very soft and thus their legs are prone to 'splaying'. If this happens, they will have to be put down. The best way to prevent this is to house them on a rough surface which gives a good grip. The rolls of corrugated cardboard used for packaging are ideal for this, but an old towel will also do.

Selling your produce

The principal quail product in this country is undoubtedly their eggs, which are almost always sold by the dozen – usually in clear or translucent plastic boxes to display the beautiful mottling. You could go further than this, however, perhaps by pre-cooking them and serving them with a little sachet of celery salt for upmarket picnics. Alternatively, you could pickle them – or even even use your imagination to make a range of miniature canapés. Indeed, I once ate a delicious hot quail starter at Heston Blumenthal's fantastic restaurant, The Fat Duck. Somehow he had managed to make a perfect Scotch egg whose inside was not only runny, but still hot.

Selling the meat of these birds is more problematic. If you are hatching and rearing your own laying birds, you will end up with a lot of unwanted males. On the Continent these are plucked and served as appetisers, but unlike Mediterranean gastronomes we seem to be put off by the very thought of eating small birds. Also, plucking is laborious and fiddly beyond belief. Some animal keepers – such as falconers and reptile owners – will buy the birds ungutted and in the feather. Ounce for ounce they then start to mount up in value, but they are so small they are still only worth a few pence each.

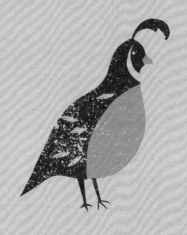

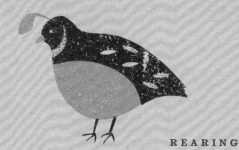

Guinea fowl

This strange-looking bird lives wild in Africa but has been domesticated for its meat. Known in French as *pintade*, its flesh has a slightly stronger taste than chicken and is not dissimilar to fresh pheasant. Despite their African origins, they are surprisingly hardy and will fly into trees at night out of the reach of predators. As a result they are one of the birds best suited to the most free-range of farming systems, where they will find the majority of their own food. If you can't afford the space, they also do well in the more usual moveable arks, where they should be fed on pheasant crumbs.

Problems

Guinea fowl are gregarious and noisy birds, chattering away to each other constantly during the day, which can cause problems with neighbours. Also, if you are an aesthete, it has to be said their bald, blue-grey, vulturine heads and necks are not exactly stunning.

Selling your produce

Although a tasty bird that is valued across the Channel, guinea fowl is not intensively farmed in Britain and so is relatively uncommon on supermarket shelves. This gives you an opportunity to side-step commercial producers. The British lack of familiarity with guinea fowl means there is a limited market for the meat, particularly given its similarity to pheasant (braces of oven-ready game birds are almost given away every autumn in traditional butchers and at the markets).

So, again, some form of processing is probably the best way of adding value to this bird. Portioning a bird is very quick and simple and it may well be worth more as its component parts than as a roaster. Creating interesting ready meals – for example, casseroles or tagines – is an alternative. Or you could cater for the summer picnic market by hot-smoking the birds and either selling them whole or shredded in a coronation-style salad.

Finally, their unusual spotted feathers could, conceivably, have a limited market in a range of arts and crafts –that is if you have the time and inclination to pluck the birds.

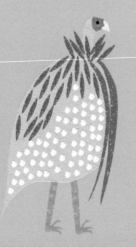

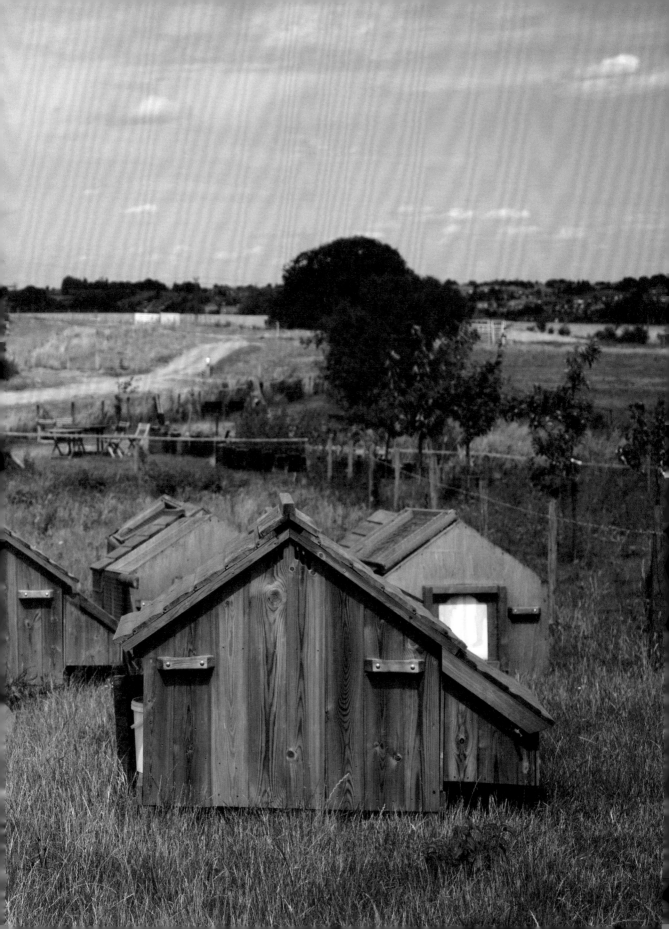

Mammals

Although most traditional British farms always had some poultry in the yard, the mainstay of our livestock agriculture has always revolved around bigger mammals. Pigs, sheep and cattle are ideally suited to living in our mild, damp climate, which makes it easier to rear well-flavoured produce.

Obviously these animals require more space than birds. Each cow, for example, will need up to an acre of grass, and while you can keep pigs on a relatively small patch of ground they will quickly turn it into a quagmire and produce a great deal of manure. Most will need some form of shelter from the elements, too (at the very least in the depths of winter) and while a little wire mesh can keep a chicken fenced in and a fox fenced out, it takes a lot more to stop a determined sheep, let alone cow or goat.

Also, while you can easily stock up poultry feeders and drinkers with a couple of days' food and ask a friend to top these up to allow you a well-deserved holiday, big animals need more attention. Yes, a cow or sheep will graze contentedly for weeks on end with no 'hands-on' care, but inevitably the moment you board the flight to the Algarve is the day they decide to break out of the paddock or gash their

foot open, so you will need a higher level of farm babysitter and will also have to be prepared to shoulder some hefty vet's bills.

The commitment in time and money is even greater if you are producing milk on a commercial basis. Come rain or shine, someone will have to be there twice a day to milk your goat, sheep or cow in a parlour which is kept scrupulously clean and is subject to regular official inspections. You will also need to work out exactly where every drop of your milk is going. It comes as a surprise to many people to discover that milk is one of the most dangerous agricultural pollutants – actually worse than slurry. The problem is that it is extremely rich in nutrients, so if it gets into a water course it will cause an explosion in algae which denudes rivers and lakes of oxygen, in turn killing any fish and handing you eye-watering fines.

To make matters more complicated, you will need a surprising amount of

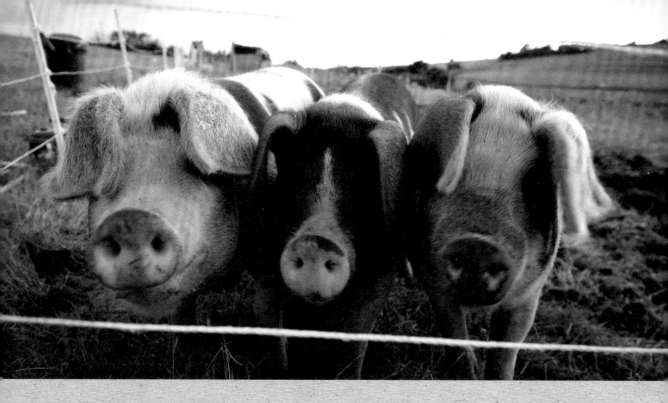

potentially expensive kit if you are intending to keep a significant amount of animals, particularly on a commercial basis; you will need at least a trailer to take them to the abattoir.

On that note, you will also need to work out where your local abattoir is and whether they are prepared to handle your choice of stock. In the old days the local butcher might have been able to deal with any livestock, but modern rules and regulations mean that even the dwindling number of small rural abattoirs which remain are increasingly specialised. Many, for example, lack the equipment needed to scald a pig, while others can cope with sheep but not goats. If you are organic, you may also need to use Soil Association-registered premises, and in many parts of the country this could involve a long drive.

If you have just a few sheep or a couple of pigs then you might be able to manage with just a four-wheel drive car or even quad bike to get around your fields, but any more than that and a tractor soon becomes necessary for lugging winter feed across snow-covered fields and to shift arks and hurdles around sodden ground.

One final consideration is all the paperwork. This isn't insurmountable, but it does take time that you need to allow for, and you may have to put up with inspections and keeping detailed records of food, medicines and movement of your animals. As a rule of thumb, the bigger the animal, the more bureaucracy there is – particularly since the outbreaks of first BSE and then foot and mouth at the turn of this century. My rule of thumb is to fill out the forms there and then so they don't get forgotten about!

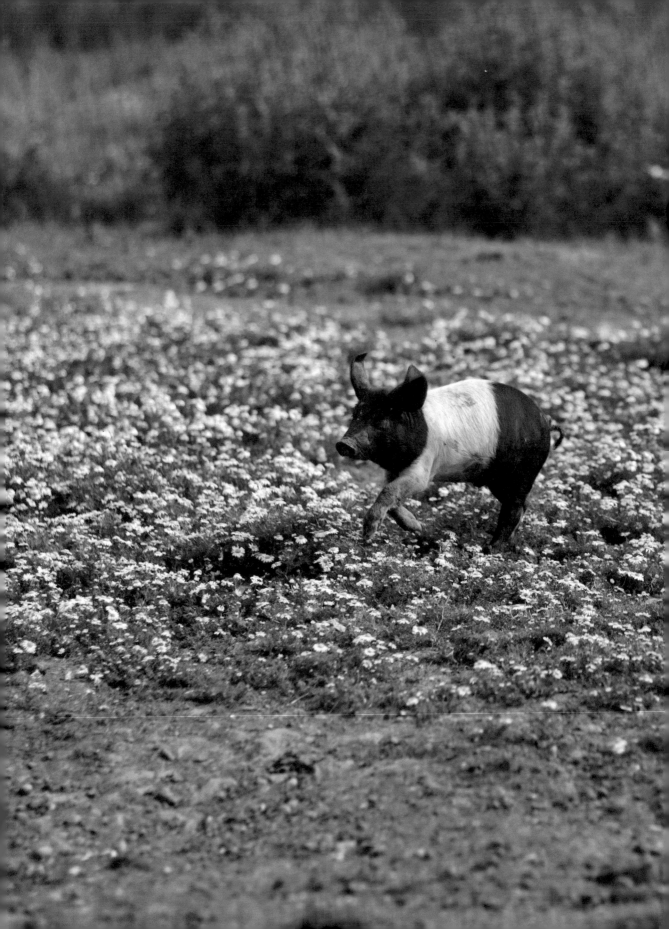

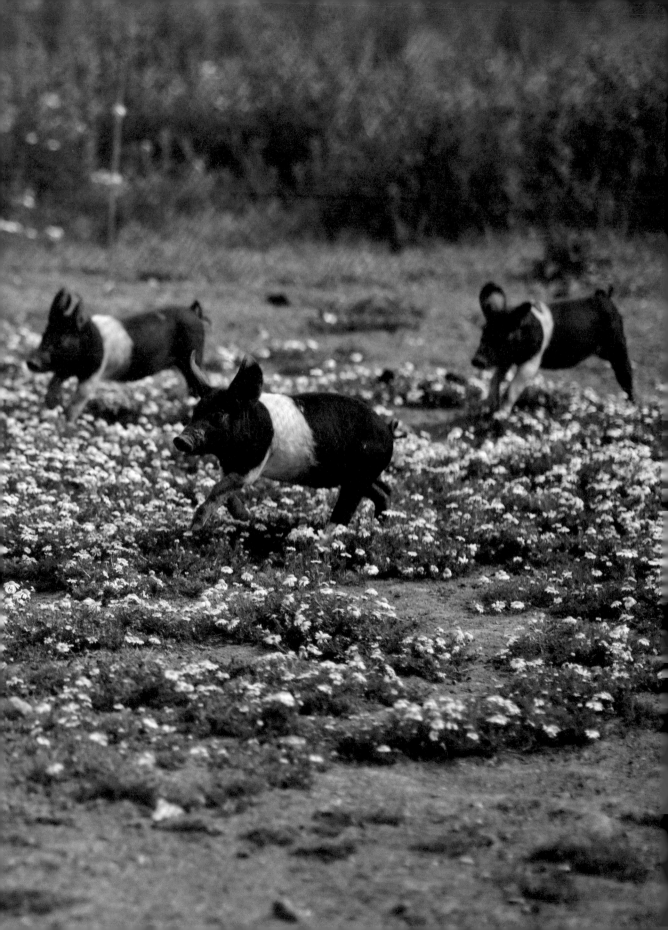

Sheep

These cloven-hoofed creatures are good converters of grass to meat, milk and wool. They have long been one of the backbones of British agriculture. During the Middle Ages the flocks that grazed the Cotswolds, Dales and Downs made millionaires out of the wool merchants that traded their fleeces and, indirectly, built the great Cistercian abbeys such as Fountains and Rievaulx. Today they are associated mainly with upland and coastal farming, thanks to their ability to cope with poor weather and rough terrain. They are fairly hardy and will do well on poor ground.

This makes them ideal for the smallholder with a large garden – although a paddock or orchard is probably better. Unlike pigs, goats or cattle, they don't need shelter from even the worst of elements (at least not if you choose one of the hardier mountain breeds). Nor do you need to provide supplementary food if you allow each enough pasture. How much depends on the breed and grazing, but you can generally put three or four ewes and their lambs on an acre of even poor ground without too much 'poaching' (over-grazing and hoof damage to the soil structure around water and added food.

You will also have to shear the older animals every year as a matter of good husbandry. Although the fleece might once have been valuable, nowadays it rarely covers the cost of shearing. The hardy native breeds that are the backbone of British sheep farming produce a very coarse yarn. Our ancestors must have had remarkably tough hides (not to mention a much more robust attitude towards body odour), because while they were prepared to wear the same woollen garments next to their skin week after week after week, today most domestic production goes to make carpets or, at best, tweed, while most of the softer wools we normally wear come from Australian or New Zealand merino sheep.

Problems

Sheep can be very frustrating. It is almost as if they start out life with a death wish; from the moment of conception they seem hell-bent on ending it all. Newborn lambs will be taken by foxes and badgers, then later on they will strangle themselves by pushing their heads through fencing, get hopelessly caught up in brambles and are often unable to get up after rolling onto their backs. All of these leave them vulnerable to crows and ravens, which have the unpleasant habit of whipping out their eyes and tongues while the poor creature lies there alive but helpless. It's only nature, of course, but it's still deeply distressing to the poor farmer.

These animals are also susceptible to a range of unpleasant diseases; some, like scab, are highly infectious and you must instantly notify the authorities if your

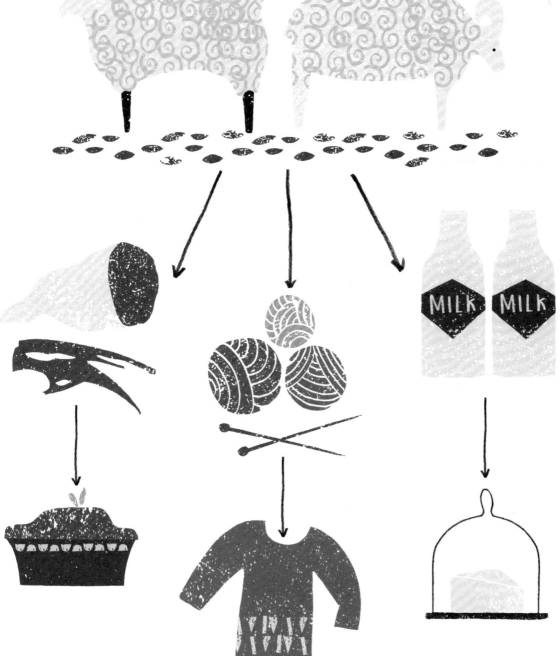

ADVANTAGES
HARDY
good on POOR GROUND
GOOD MARKET
for MEAT

DISADVANTAGES
WOOL No longer
VALUABLE
DISEASES
Troublesome

MILK MILK

flock is infected. In damp conditions sheep readily pick up foot rot (a fungal disease which makes them limp), and they also attract ticks, worms and fly strike – where carnivorous flies lay their eggs in the dirty fleece around the backside and then the maggots eat their way into the thighs. As a result, you will need to keep a close eye on your stock even at quiet times of the year and regularly worm and clip off any dung (or 'dags') clinging to their rear ends.

They might not be quite the most heavily regulated farm livestock, but plenty of paperwork goes with each flock of sheep, whatever its size. This has only gone up since the outbreaks of foot and mouth in 2001 and 2007 – and blue tongue disease.

Breeds

British sheep are usually split into two broad camps: lowland and mountain. The former are less hardy but bigger. Until recently the supermarkets insisted British consumers were only interested in larger cuts, so these were the only ones to appear in most chilled cabinets. Meanwhile, the smaller mountain breeds were exported live to Continental markets (bizarrely, an animal is deemed to have come from where it is killed, so Scottish lambs might be driven all the way to Greece to be slaughtered and then sold as 'local').

The important thing to remember is that each traditional breed was developed for a purpose – and this usually included coping with specific climate and landscape requirements. Thus a good tip when choosing your stock is to check which breeds are popular with your neighbours and follow their example (or at least ask for suggestions).

Suffolk: A big meat-producing breed (rams 110–160kg; ewes 80–110kg), this is often crossed with a hardier, but smaller, mountain breed to get a mule which combines the virtues of both breeds.

Scottish Blackface: The most common breed in Britain (almost one in three sheep here is a Blackface), this is a tough mountain breed with a long coat that has been bred to withstand the rigours of life outside in a Highland winter.

Jacob: An ancient breed which in some ways is more like a goat than a sheep. The rams can have up to six horns, and despite several thousand years of domestication, as a breed it appears relatively unimproved over this time and still very similar to its wild European ancestors. This rare-breed animal is relatively small, hardy and produces a multi-coloured wool, all of which make it popular among hobby farmers.

Lacaune: Almost all the world's Roquefort cheese comes from this breed. It is France's most popular dairy sheep and can yield up to 280 litres per lactation.

Merino: Originally developed in medieval Spain, this is now the great Australian meat and wool breed. Although most of the wool used in clothing today comes from this breed, it likes warm weather and so it struggles with our climate.

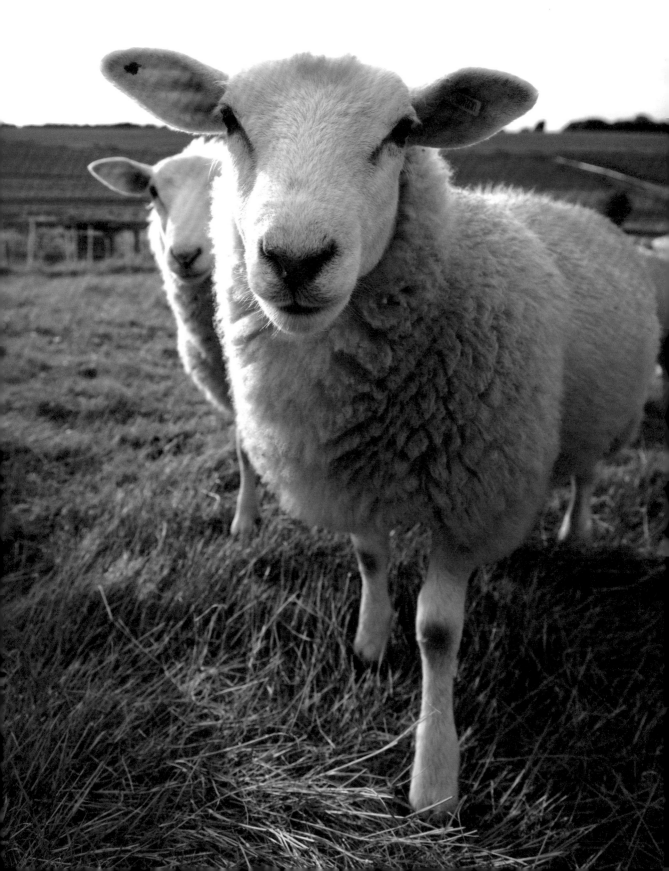

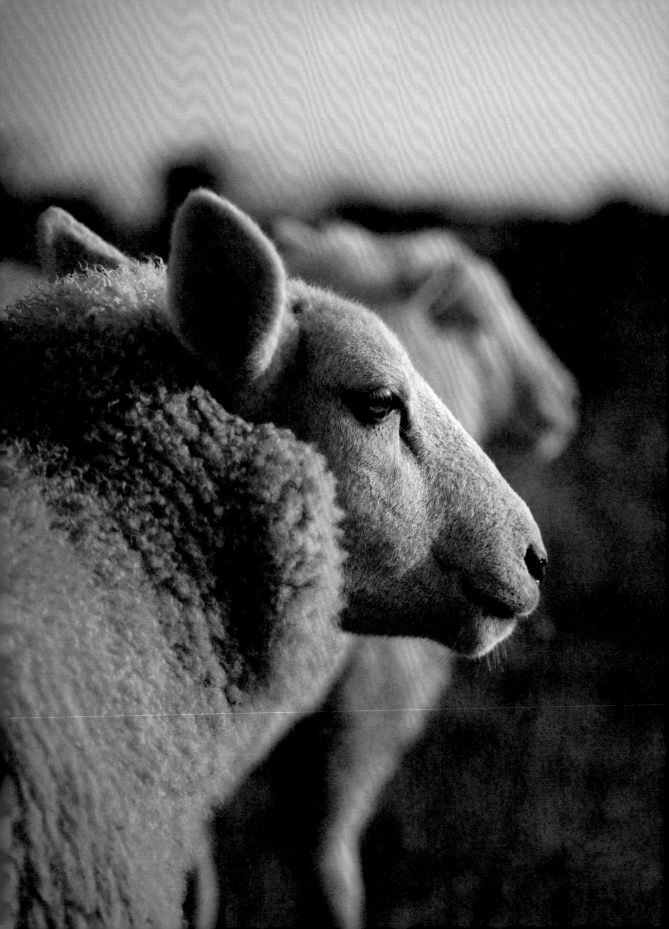

Selling your produce

Sheep produce good-quality meat and fleeces for which there is a ready market. In addition, some smallholders are starting to produce 'organically tanned' hides and others are finding uses for the horns – which can be softened with heat and shaped or carved to make walking stick handles or traditional crooks. In fact, given the huge growth in the popularity of extendable walking poles among hikers, this could well be an interesting market. In many parts of the world they are also kept as dairy animals, and although this is still comparatively unusual in Britain, there is a market for the milk, most of which becomes cheese.

As an established staple meat, almost all lamb is sold in the familiar cuts of shoulder, neck, belly, chops and legs (plus, of course, liver and kidneys). However, there is still scope for bumping up your margins with a bit of imaginative butchery. A rack of lamb may be little more than an unseparated row of chops, but many customers are happy to pay significantly more for it – particularly if you sell it complete with those little paper hats to dress the rib ends and a big bunch of fresh rosemary or a home-made mint sauce. Similarly, although the shoulder is arguably a better roasting joint than the leg, modern consumers are put off by the large flat shoulder blade. You can not only get round this by removing it, but in the process you create a cavity which you can fill with a fresh herb stuffing or interesting spice or even fruit mix. Likewise, the already prime leg cut can also be boned to create a 'butterfly' (perfect marinated and chargrilled on a barbecue). As with so many carcasses, some cuts can be difficult to sell because of the high fat content, but the same vice also makes them perfect for burgers, kofte kebabs and even sausages.

Another interesting take is to branch into mutton (see the case study on the next page) or to market lamb by tying it tightly to its origins. Many chefs now rate Welsh lamb, for example, as the best in the world, while others are working hard to promote salt marsh and Shetland seaweed brands. Similarly, Lakeland sheep, once threatened with extinction by foot and mouth, have been thrown a lifeline by farmers who are now promoting their 'hefted' upbringing (the ewes wander freely across the unfenced hills, each teaching their lambs to stay within their traditional territory).

CASE STUDY >>

CASE STUDY The Mutton Entrepreneur

Tony DAVIES is an UNLIKELY revolutionary. His family has farmed the HENFRON in MID Wales for 160 years and he is FIERCELY proud of his ROOTS.

Even today he prefers to round up his flocks on horseback rather than the more usual quad, and although English is his native tongue he uses Welsh commands to work his dogs. Yet over the past five years this 45-year-old traditionalist has launched an assault on the nation's eating habits. He believes it is time we were reintroduced to the joys of mutton and in the process has carved himself a profitable niche.

At first glance his determination to return to the past and switch production from young lambs to old sheep seems foolhardy. To begin with, most people have never tasted mutton. For years even good butchers – let alone modern supermarkets – refused to believe this meat had a market. Most people would be hard-pressed to define the word (mutton means a sheep over two years, lamb is less than 12 months and a 'hogget' straddles the difference).

Tony was convinced this ignorance does the meat a grave disservice. After all, for centuries mutton was central to the British diet (take a look at classic literature where characters are forever calling for mutton chops as they arrive at coaching inns). Lamb – like all 'young' meats – was reserved for the rich.

This explains why mutton went so quickly out of fashion when cheap imports of New Zealand lamb began to flood into the country during the 1950s and 1960s. Our eating habits have always been class-conscious, so the nation switched en masse to the 'exclusive' product, even though it lacks the superior

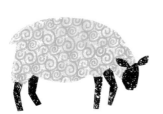

flavour and texture of older animals. British farmers were not far behind, and by the 1970s virtually all hill farms had switched their production from mutton to lambs.

As a result, when Tony announced he was reverting to the inter-wars farming practised by his grandfather, he was greeted with hoots of derision from his neighbours who failed to spot the sound rationale behind his business plan.

The most important prompt was a change in agricultural subsidies. Until early this century farmers were paid a 'headage' for every ewe they kept. This encouraged them to keep as many breeding ewes as possible. The wethers (male lambs) were sold in late summer and farmers would buy in extra food to support as many ewes as possible over the winter. This prompted over-stocking and over-grazing to the detriment of the uplands, so in 2004 subsidies were switched to an acreage basis.

Unlike most of his neighbours, Tony spotted that traditional farming was actually more suited to the new system. 'Before the war my grandfather would have kept wethers [castrated males] until they were three or four years old and much bigger than today's six-month-old lambs,' he says. 'In those days the farm revolved around the number of animals the land could support in winter.'

Tony spotted this would work well with the new subsidy regime and now the Henfron flock contains far more males with an older average age than before, and because wethers are hardier than lambing ewes they can be kept out all year. This means Tony is now virtually self-sufficient in feed (he makes some hay, but no longer needs to buy in winter food from outside).

Better still, he was able to convert to organic at very little cost: 'I'd expected it to be difficult and involve some costly changes, but it turns out we were already complying with – or even exceeding – almost all of the rules,' he says. The major difference is he now has to keep records to prove he is doing what he has always done and must consult a vet before treating any of his animals.

His new farming approach also has great environmental benefits for his land. Low-level winter grazing stops the delicate upland grazing from becoming too matted, yet reduced stocking means there is less 'poaching' (trampling damage to the soil, particularly around feeding stations). This has greatly benefited the farm's wildflower meadows, many of which are listed as Sites of Special Scientific Interest (SSSIs) – something that Tony has exploited in his marketing material.

This quiet revolution in the hills does, of course, require consumers to rediscover the traditional taste for mutton, but again it seems Tony was ahead of the game when it came to spotting a trend. Within just a few months of launching the Elan Valley Mutton Company, many TV chefs and even Prince Charles were championing the virtues of mutton as a versatile meat, and a fashion for the unfashionable had begun.

Goats

Goats are a good animal for the smallholder. They have the potential to be a wonderful triple-purpose creature, capable of producing meat, milk and wool. They are certainly a mainstay of small-scale farming in many other parts of the world, but are largely missing from British agriculture. Or rather, their presence as a feral animal in parts of Wales and the West Country, plus a few Scottish islands, shows they once played a part here, but generally our farmers have preferred sheep. There is no real reason why this should be the case. In Greece, Spain, and even France, goats are popular for both their meat and perhaps even more for their milk.

Perhaps the reason for their lack of popularity is that they are rather more sensitive than sheep. So they will need protection in winter, and if they are to kid well, the does will need supplementary feeding with a high-quality concentrate such as oats or fodder beet.

Benefits

Goats grow quickly to produce a red meat which is low in fat. In a health-conscious age, this means goat is increasingly being promoted as a better alternative to lamb or beef. Similarly, although the milk is comparable to that of a cow, many people find it more digestible, and because the fat globules are smaller these separate out less easily, meaning it doesn't require homogenising. Despite this, the milk makes excellent butter (which is particularly white, owing to the structure of the fat) and also cheeses, such as feta and a huge variety of 'chevres' (actually just French for 'goat').

Goats love rough ground and can thrive where other livestock would struggle. While they will graze, in general they prefer to browse on scrub, and as creatures whose ancestors came from mountainous areas most breeds are sure-footed and thrive in tough terrain. As a result some charities promote them as a development tool for emerging economies, and in this country several Wildlife Trusts use them as unpaid ground staff on awkward reserves such as Betchworth Quarry in Surrey and Devon's Valley of the Rocks.

One final attraction is the undoubted intelligence and feisty natures of these animals. Each has a distinct character of its own and this can make them great fun to be with.

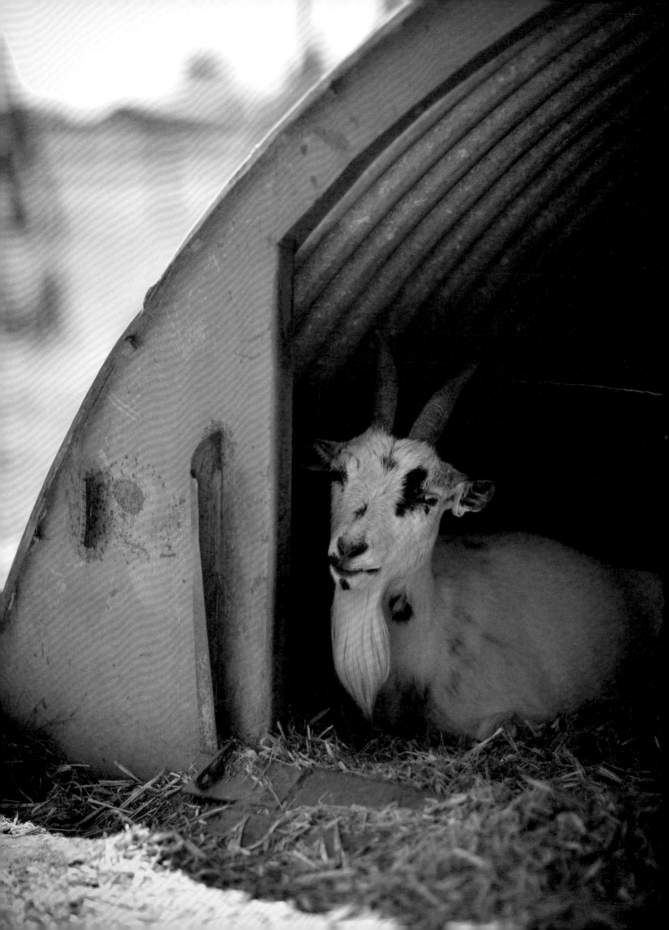

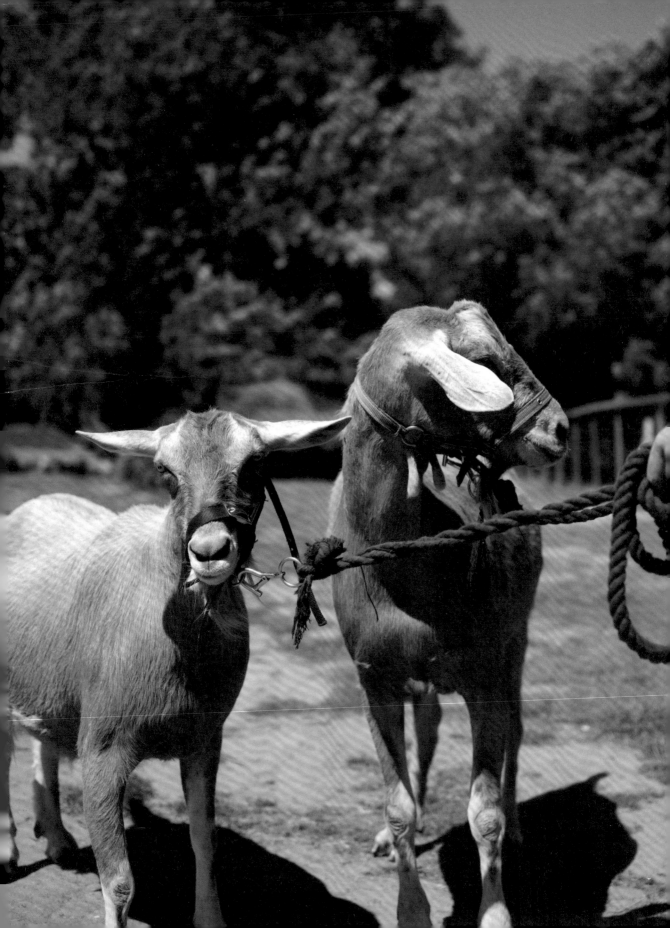

Problems

As so often, the downsides of goats are usually simply the other side of the benefit coin. As large mammals, they need a fair amount of space so are not really suitable for a back garden. This is particularly true because while they will nibble at grass, if that's all that's going, they much prefer to browse and so will make a bee-line for the herbaceous border, fruit bushes and vegetable patch rather than stay on the lawn. They can devastate trees, hedges, fruit bushes or the vegetable patch in a matter of minutes and if they get anywhere near plants you care about you will very quickly recognise why they are dubbed 'the desert-maker' in many parts of the world.

In other words, wherever you put goats, you will need to keep them very tightly controlled. This can be difficult, however, because they are mountain creatures. For many people the answer is tethering; others turn to electric fencing; while really good conventional mesh and barbed wire can also work. Even so, some are consummate escapologists and if (or rather when) they do, you or your neighbours will soon know about it.

This destructive drive is linked to their nutritional requirements. It takes the consumption of a lot of high-quality vegetation for any animal to make meat or milk. Cows and sheep can do this on good grass, but goats are built to feed on woodier matter and so many – but particularly the dairy breeds – crave shrubs and will do anything to get to them.

If you want to milk your animals, you not only have to be prepared to commit to twice-daily milking, but work out exactly where your produce is going. Each nanny will give up to four litres of milk a day, which is too much for most families to consume in liquid form. This means you either have to change it into cheese or butter, or sell it. All these options are certainly possible, but they are yet another level of commitment, and if you are selling to a shop or the public you will need expensive bottling and labelling equipment. Also, don't forget that each nanny only produces milk for about nine months of the year, so your customers will have to cope with a varying supply.

The other by-product of dairy goats, of course, is offspring. Each lactation results in one and three kids. If you have the space the females can join your milking herd, but some will be male and will either have to be put down at birth or reared for meat (in which case they need to be castrated to reduce their gaminess).

Breeds

As one might expect of a farm animal with a near-global distribution, there are a wide range of goat sizes and temperaments so you need to do your research to decide which is best for your needs and space. European breeds tend to be bigger and intended primarily as dairy animals, while those from hot climates (where milk quickly goes off) are more likely to be for meat, or sometimes their fleece.

Angora: This breed originally comes from Turkey, but it is now farmed all over the world for its fleece. Does are shorn twice a year to yield a total of 5–8kg of the long lustrous fibres we know as mohair.

Alpine: This dairy breed was developed in the French Alps, and with does weighing up to 60kg the animals are comparatively large. Alpine goats are inveterate escapologists and will leap over surprisingly tall fences if they decide something on the other side looks particularly edible.

Anglo-Nubian: A dual-purpose breed with Middle Eastern origins, it has large pendulous ears and is well suited to life in hotter climates. Although the doe's milk yield is not as great as some other dairy breeds, she will weigh over 60kg and so makes a good all-round animal.

Boer: As the name suggests, this was originally developed in South Africa (boer means 'farmer' in Afrikaans). This is an attractive white and orange breed which is relatively docile and easy to contain. The goats produce very good meat, but the carcass is comparatively small, so 'bucks' are often crossed with bigger dairy breeds to get the confirmation of the father and the size of the female.

Selling your produce

Although there is certainly a market for the meat, milk is probably the easiest goat product to sell.

The best way to maximise on the value of any milk is almost certainly to turn it into cheese. Traditionally this was how people stored the glut of summer milk for the winter months, but today we think of cheese more as an upmarket product. Certainly making cheese can increase the value of the raw material, milk, several fold.

Even if Britain has little in the way of a goat-farming tradition, most people are very familiar with the cheese and so it has a ready market. Fortunately, it is also relatively simple to make a range of soft and hard cheeses from goat's milk, and once you know what you are doing you can customise the recipe to create a unique product (for example by wrapping the cheese in leaves or including home-grown herbs or spices). If this is for your own consumption and not for sale, you can do this in a kitchen, but if you intend to sell it you will need proper facilities and you will have to keep scrupulously to hygiene regulations. Softer cheeses of the type generally sold as chevre are simpler and quicker to make than the hard varieties; they also require less specialist equipment and long-term storage.

The meat is potentially a little more problematic because most people in this country are unfamiliar with it. This can deter many customers, while those that are brave enough to experiment may need a little educating. Goat has much less fat than its apparent look-alike, lamb, and consequently it has a tendency to dry out when cooked; the last thing you want is for a new customer to get things wrong and to decide it is a tough and unpleasant product. As with anything, you should be aiming for that first purchase to be just the start of a long-term relationship.

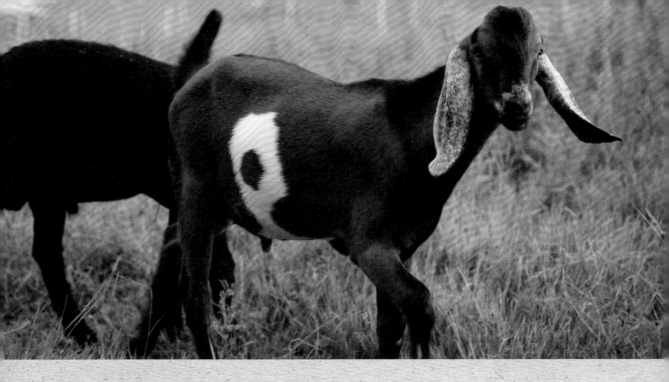

There is, however, a great demand for the meat from many of the ethnic groups that have settled here over the past half century – particularly those from the Indian subcontinent and the Caribbean. There are big ethnic markets in many of the major cities in Britain, but these customers present a very different challenge. They will probably simply want cuts and, as with any carcass, you may find you have the problem of some cuts (probably the 'prime' legs and saddle) being far more popular than the cheaper flesh from the shoulders, neck and belly. Fortunately, the same fattier cuts are easy to turn into sausages – which can also make the best introduction for less-experienced customers. One possibility would be to play on goat's associations with spicy cuisines and produce a range of spicy Caribbean, African or Indian recipes. An alternative is to produce

a range of ready meals – which again largely circumnavigates the problem of customer ignorance.

Finally, don't forget the rest of the animal. If you are really determined you can wash the intestines out either to make your own sausage casings or even 'cat gut' (most instrument strings are actually not feline but goat). However, the skin is a more realistic by-product, which can be woven to make a good wall hanging or rug – although the animal's pungent musky smell can be difficult to eradicate completely. The wool from some breeds, of course – notably the Angora – is also very highly prized by knitters and can fetch high prices.

When it is defoliated the skin makes a durable, soft leather (as in kid gloves). Indeed, some breeds have actually been developed for their hides, with the meat and milk being the by-products.

FENCING THEM IN

Unless you have 'hefted' flocks (unfenced sheep which are taught the farm boundaries by their mothers and which are only rounded up once or twice a year), you will need to restrain your animals. It is vital to keep them in one place and protect them from predators, but also to protect crops and avoid rows with neighbours. It can also be very expensive because of the lengths of boundary involved: after all, even a modest garden probably has a 50–100-yard perimeter, while a five-acre smallholding could easily contain half a mile of fencing.

✔ GO ELECTRIC

This is a brilliant way of containing livestock. It's cheap, portable and quick to put up, which means you can regularly move your animals around a field, giving them fresh grazing, while reducing 'poaching' (hoof damage to the ground) and reducing parasite build-ups. It works well with most livestock, provided the right 'barrier' is used. This means one or two strands of wire for pigs, netting for sheep and tape for horses and cattle. Netting is also useful with poultry, but here its main use is to keep out marauding foxes rather than keep in the birds.

Broadly speaking electric fencing has one of two power sources: mains and battery. Both work on the same principle of creating a very high-voltage, low-ampage, DC output. One terminal connects to the boundary wire while the other is earthed. When an animal touches the wire the current earths down its leg to create a circuit back to the unit. This voltage gives an unpleasant jolt (usually accompanied by a little 'crack!'), which is entirely harmless. Using a mains supply is ridiculously cheap because it uses almost no electricity and you can run literally miles of fencing from one unit, but this is much less adaptable than the alternative.

In the old days portable units were chunky affairs which needed a lot of muscle to lug around. Today some are about the size of a mug, with the current coming from a couple of standard 'D' torch batteries (if you really want to save money and the planet you can use rechargeables). These little units are capable of running up to 250 metres of fencing for a month or two before the batteries need replacing.

There are two minor issues with electric fencing, however. Most livestock needs to learn to respect electricity. If you put a frisky or scared animal in a field with a strand of electricity between it and whatever it thinks it wants, it is likely to barge straight through the barrier. Yes, it may get a shock as it goes, but it is as likely to jump onto the other side as stay in its enclosure. The solution is to train your animals by confining them in an escape-proof barn or field with the wire around the perimeter. Brushing against the wires for a couple of days they will learn this is best avoided. Once trained they will happily stay behind the fencing, even when the batteries have accidentally run out of juice.

Grass and branches are the other problem. As plants grow and brush against the wire, they create a short-circuit which rapidly drains the battery. The answer is simple: you need to regularly walk along the line with a brush cutter, chopping back the foliage.

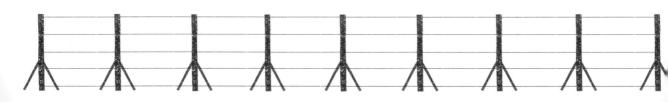

✓ KEEP IT CONVENTIONAL

Post-and-rail fencing looks good and is generally fine for horses and donkeys, but it won't contain most other livestock. Sheep, goats and pigs will squeeze through or under, while a determined cow intent on juicy vegetation on the other side will push it over. In most cases wire and posts give the quickest and cheapest way of creating a permanent stock-proof barrier. Horses can be restrained merely with a few strands of taut wire (think of railway fencing). This avoids accidental scratches to both them and you, but cattle will push hard so generally require barbed wire. Sheep and goats are even more persistent and ingenious, thus they need netting along the bottom with a strand of wire along the top. Plain wire will do, but barbed wire is more effective, particularly for determined escape artists like the livelier goats and mountain sheep. Most people use heavy-gauge square mesh, but if rabbits are a problem, more expensive chicken wire can sometimes keep them out (although in my experience it rarely does). The lighter wire doesn't last as long as heavier-gauge material, which should survive for 30 years unless people regularly clamber over it (in which case a stile can save a lot of money in the long term).

The big challenge, however, is to keep the wire and netting taut. The slightest sag and your stocks' eyes will light up like Steve McQueen in *The Great Escape*: a small push, heave or squeeze and they will be rampaging through your vegetable garden. To tighten everything up, you need either a good four-wheel drive to pull it taut or a special hand crank (in other words you can't simply rely on your own weight). I can't stress enough that to work the thing has to be as tight as a guitar string, so ideally you should put it up on a hot summer's day when the wire is at its greatest expansion (this will leave it even tighter in winter when the stock are most determined to find more food). For it to stay taut, however, you should pay particular attention to the corner posts where all the strains are concentrated. This means using larger posts supported with sturdy stays, driven hard in the ground at a 45-degree angle and hammered tight into the upright.

Provided the wire is tight, posts and stakes are easily the fence's weakest link. While galvanised wire will last for decades as long as it is not touching the soil, decay starts as soon as the wood goes into the ground. How long they stay strong depends on whether they have been treated, their diameter and the timber. 'Treatment' (rot-proofing) is most critical. This can extend a stake's life by a factor of four or five at the cost of only a few pence each. The type of timber used is important too. Oak, for example, lasts much longer than spruce. In an exposed wet spot untreated softwood disintegrates within two to five years, while treated could hope for 10–20 years. Oak should last double this, but commercial hardwood stakes can be very expensive. If you are happy for your fences to have a rustic appearance, you can often source your own for free – or buy them from someone who is coppicing or hedging. They may retain their bark and not be dead straight, but they will be cheap. If this isn't possible, get hold of the 'red' softwoods (like larch, Douglas fir and Scots pine). Their sap contains natural preservatives so their life-expectancy is comparable to oak, which can be several decades if properly treated.

The greater the diameter, the longer it takes to rot through. Resist the temptation to use 'halves' or 'quarters' (stakes which have been cut lengthways). This might produce a cheaper upright, but it reduces its strength and increases the surface area in contact with the soil.

If you must economise, use the new high-tensile netting which has more spring in it, allowing you to put bigger spaces between the stakes. Provided you use really sound posts, supported with good stays, you can put staves in at 20- rather than 10-metre spacings.

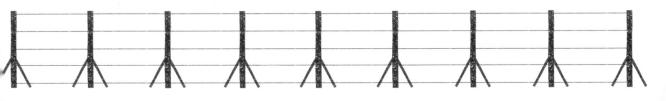

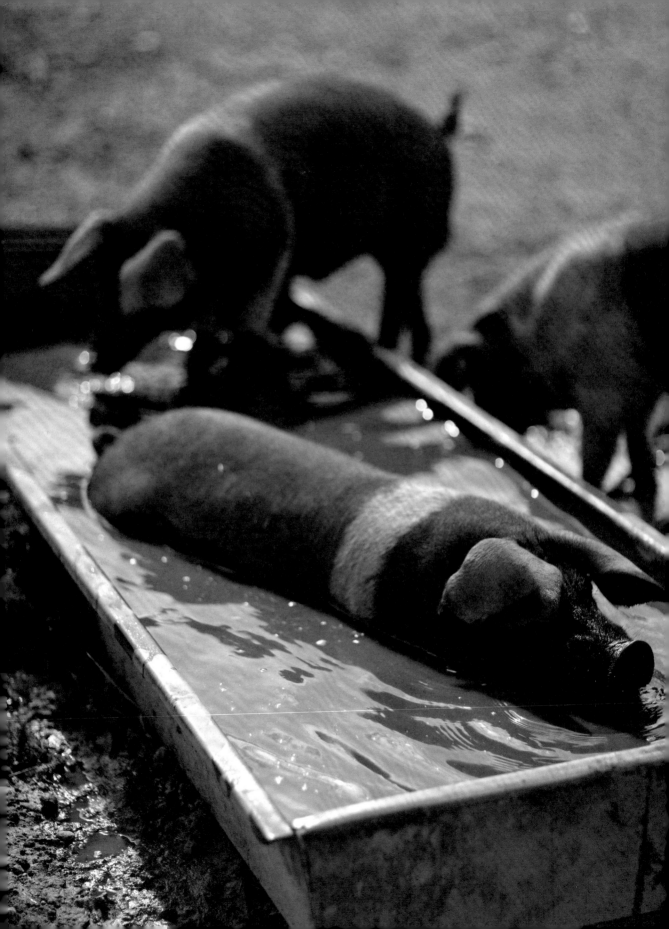

Pigs

There are very good reasons why these lovable animals play a central role in Asian, Polynesian, African and European farming cultures. Their omnivorous diet is key to this – they can be reared on almost anything and are adept at finding their own food. In many parts of the world they roam freely around towns and villages, acting as unpaid refuse collectors.

Here in Britain during the Middle Ages our ancestors used to rear them on 'pannage' – using boys to drive them into the ancient forests where they would grow during the summer by snuffling through the leaf mould to find bulbs and grubs, before finally being fattened on the rich autumn acorn harvest. Later, most cottagers would have a sty at the end of the garden where the pig would act as a living waste-disposal unit, turning garden trimmings and kitchen scraps into pork and bacon.

Thanks to health and hygiene regulations, things are a bit more complicated today, but pigs are still an attractive option for the would-be farmer and food producer. They can still be kept in traditional walled sties with an outdoor yard, but my preference is certainly for outdoor ranging behind electric fencing. They are naturally social animals, so the weaners should be allowed to wander around together with a few communal shelters provided. Breeding sows should be given individual enclosures, however, where they can rear their young without disturbance from other adults.

You will need to feed your pigs every day with a balanced diet that contains the correct level of protein, but the animals will supplement their diet with wild foods throughout the summer and autumn months if allowed to free range. If you are lucky enough to have access to some mature oak woodland you can recreate the pannage system. This can actually be good for the forest floor, because as they snuffle through the leaf mould they eat weeds and create a natural seed bed. That said, you can have too much of a good thing. They feed naturally by rooting in the soil, so unless you move them frequently or let them roam very widely, they will inevitably chew up the ground and turn it into a ploughed field.

A pig is a happy, active creature, and should be allowed to run around and enjoy the open air just on principle. Also, if you intend to rear pigs as a commercial venture, it is important to bear in mind that you won't be able to put a premium price on your meat unless they have built up some muscle tone and your customers will also expect you to operate to the highest welfare standards. In fact, these will almost certainly be an important part of your marketing, so you must give your pigs plenty of room, move them onto fresh land regularly and preferably have them somewhere where your customers can see them looking happy and healthy.

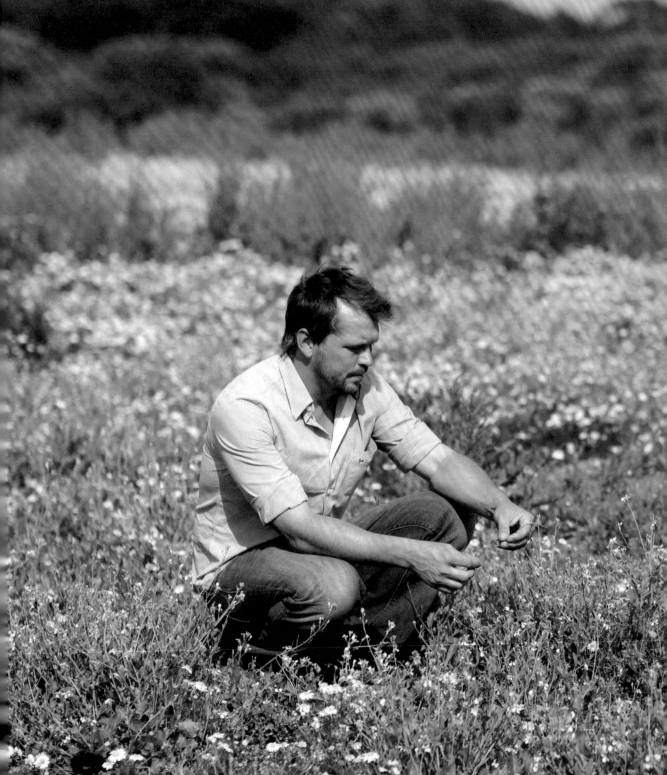

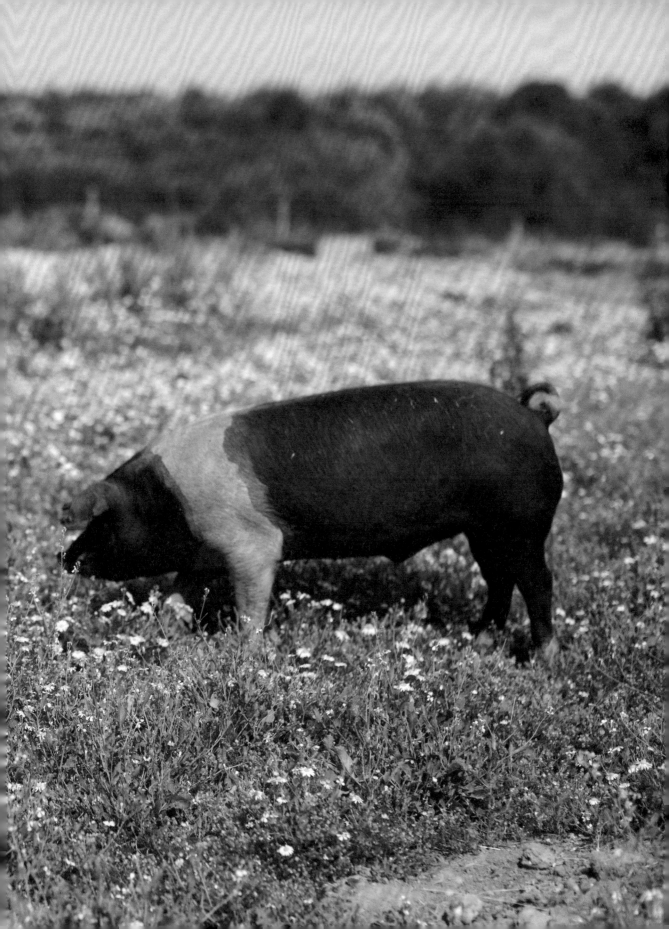

Pigs are also easy to keep. Assuming they are living outdoors (which hugely reduces mucking out) in the process they will rotovate and fertilise the land they are on. As I've said, they do need feeding every day but will find a lot of their own food – if you give them enough space – eating grass and rooting in the ground for slugs, worms and insects, which will reduce your feed bills. You will need to make sure they have plenty of fresh water, too. If you train pigs properly, they are easy to confine with electric fencing, which is cheap and flexible – again representing a huge cost saving. If you house them in a lightweight ark you can move them around your land, confining them if you want them to dig it up, or giving them plenty of space and moving the fences regularly if you want them to find most of their own food without churning up the pasture.

Pigs are unusually productive for large creatures. At three months, three weeks and three days, their gestation period is fairly short compared to cattle, or even sheep. They have large litters too; while other livestock usually have just one calf or lamb (twins, if you're lucky), a sow can produce up to 17 piglets in a litter (although we aim for 8–10 because we use traditional breeds). The piglets are quick to mature, too, with the young ready for slaughter at about six months (modern commercial hybrids are ready at five), while the gilts (young sows) are fertile at about the same age.

They are also generally very healthy – which means your vet's bills should be low. For example, unlike many larger forms of livestock, piglets are the perfect shape for easy birthing. Calves and lambs have long legs, which have an irritating habit of getting in the way, but piglets are effectively little torpedoes, so the sow rarely needs help. Instead she just fires out her litter, often in a matter of a few minutes, allowing you to sit back and watch the show.

Pigs are also great fun – which has to be a major plus. If I want to unwind, I spend time watching the cattle; it's a great way to relax and calm down. But if I want fun, I visit the pigs. They have such a huge range of personalities; some take life slowly, lying down and sunbathing, while others are constantly curious, rooting around and investigating. They can also be really affectionate and they're intelligent, too – which makes them all the more endearing.

Problems

There are downsides, of course. Some pigs will just graze and cause very little damage, but others seem to have a sonar-like ability to spot grubs and larvae deep below ground. Then they just go down and down, ploughing their way into the soil and leaving the field looking like Passchendaele. This can be great if you want to turn over rough ground, but it has its problems, too. By exposing bare soil (which is also heavily manured) they create the perfect seed bed for weeds such as thistles, docks, nettles, fat hen and

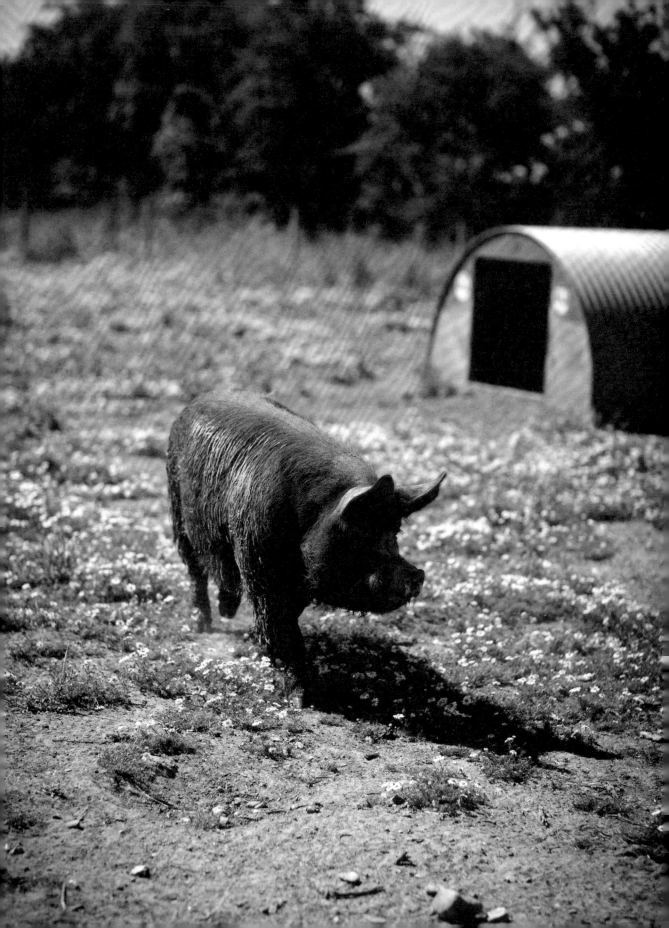

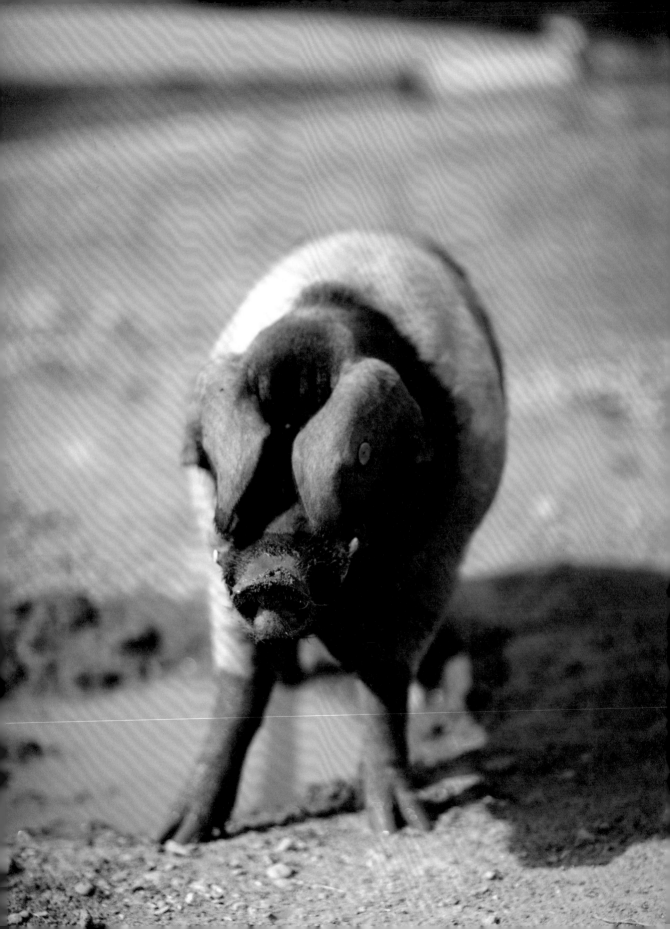

chickweed. This means you have to act fast after you take the pigs off the land; either sow it with another crop or grass ley, or move in other animals, such as goats or Soay sheep.

The combination of two very different animals works well, with the sheep – which are natural browsers – acting as unpaid weeding machines, turning the docks and thistles into tasty rare-breed meat. We did this with a patch of rough ground, using pigs to churn it up, then moving in Soay sheep, then pigs again, before finally sowing it with grass and moving in cattle.

Breeds

Traditional breeds are part of our heritage. I can never understand why we instinctively put a value on paintings and jewellery, fill museums with artefacts from the past and yet do not view rare breeds in the same light – they are just as much a part of our history. Each breed was developed over hundreds of years to suit local circumstances. The Tamworth, for example, is one of the oldest breeds and is a descendant of the wild boar which once roamed Britain's woods, bearing very few of the Asian genes that give the fast-growing qualities to most commercial breeds. The Gloucester Old Spots, on the other hand, was developed to eat grass in the cider orchards of the West Country before being fattened on the windfalls in autumn.

There is more to traditional breeds than sentimentality, though. Most have thicker bristles than modern commercial hybrids, which makes them hardier and less susceptible to sunburn (although this can be a problem at some abattoirs). Also, while they are slower growing than commercial hybrids, this results in denser muscle fibre, which gives the meat a superior texture. Another benefit is that the flesh contains more fat. This might sound strange to a cholesterol-obsessed generation, but the fat melts and bastes the meat as it cooks, resulting in a better flavour. Most chefs and discerning diners recognise that this makes for a superior ingredient.

Not that there is anything wrong with modern hybrids; most commercial pigs are based on the fast-growing white Landrace, which was originally developed by crossing European breeds with animals from Asia. They are more prolific, producing bigger litters which grow quickly, being ready for slaughter at just five months old, while my pigs take seven months to reach killing weight to produce a carcass which fits in perfectly with most twenty-first-century needs. Something like 98 per cent of the pork and bacon we eat comes from these, so they are clearly an excellent breed for modern times. If you are a farmer trying to supply the big supermarkets in what must be one of the most competitive meat markets in Europe, there is no alternative to these hybrids. In general, however, small producers are much better off focusing on a traditional breed to create an unusual top-quality meat which can then be sold at a premium.

There are a score of ancient varieties, each of which has its own unique qualities, but I stock six on my farm because these seem particularly suited to my needs. Broadly I need animals that are slow-enough growing to produce a superior meat, yet still be commercially viable. I also want a range of shapes for different purposes – the less fatty breeds are better for pork while the plumper animals make better bacon and sausages.

Tamworth: These rusty, prick-eared pigs must be one of the prettiest breeds and are also tame and friendly (which can be important for marketing and on farms which encourage visitors). They are a really ancient breed, perfected on a Staffordshire estate by Sir Robert Peel, the nineteenth-century Prime Minister and inventor of the modern police force. These are reputed to make the best bacon, but in my experience their litters can be small, struggling to get over six or so.

Gloucester Old Spots: Originally developed to live in West Country cider orchards, this breed has grown in number and is now one of the most numerous traditional breeds. It is an excellent dual-purpose pig, producing wonderful pork and excellent bacon. The sows also make great mothers and often produce good-sized litters.

Saddleback: This was developed by mixing Wessex and Essex breeds to produce an attractive piebald animal. These are also great dual-purpose pigs and ideal for me because of the East Anglian connection, which makes them easy to market locally.

Middle white: Not to be confused with the commercial long white (which is descended from the Landrace), this is primarily a pork pig with a relatively low fat content (for a traditional pig). Perhaps because of this it is highly valued in Japan.

Berkshire: This attractive black pig was reputedly discovered by Cromwellian troops during the English Civil War as they besieged the king in his Oxford headquarters. It is another porker with a delicate and relatively fast-maturing meat which means it is sometimes called the 'lady's pig'. It is also arguably the most famous literary breed, playing a starring role as the Empress of Blandings in P.G. Wodehouse's classic Blandings Castle series and as Napoleon in Orwell's *Animal Farm.*

Large black: These have lovely big ears which make them look as if they are wearing sunglasses. They are great for crossing with other breeds, and although they are really a porker, we also use them for bacon, cutting the rind off fat animals and inserting loads of rosemary and thyme into the lard so that when it's sliced there is a lovely ring of herbs around the meat: perfect fried for breakfast and served with a lovely fresh duck egg.

Wild boar: These have been farmed here as a novelty meat since the 1960s. At first glance the fact that their meat retails for three or four times the price of conventional pork makes them seem very attractive, but as usual there is a good reason for this. Officially they are a dangerous wild animal, so you need a special licence to keep them (although

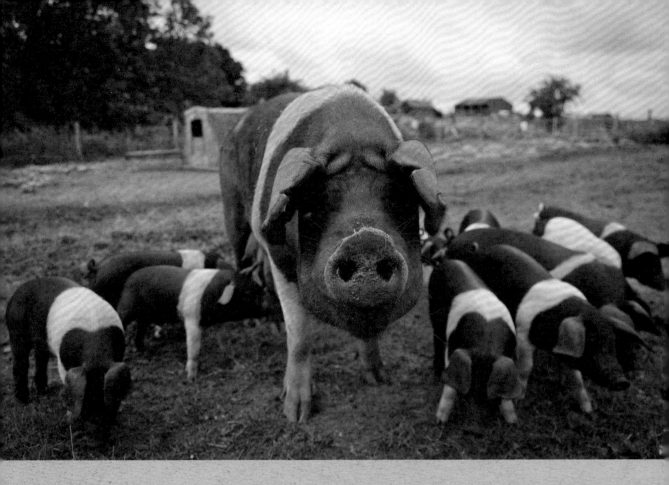

this regulation may soon change). They are certainly extremely powerful and the adults have razor-sharp tusks which can inflict serious injury, and they are fantastic escape artists, and once out they are almost impossible to catch (which explains why Britain's feral boar population is currently estimated to be thousands strong). Wild boar are also unbelievably slow-growing, not reaching killing weight until they are 18 months old. That said, some farmers have had great success with them, but they are not really for beginners. If you want to go into wild boar, my advice would be to start with a traditional breed and then branch out once you have a few years' experience.

Selling your produce

I love my pigs, but, to be hard-nosed, they are particularly wonderful because, unlike other big meat-producing animals, they lend themselves to an unusually large range of products. Beef and lamb are rarely much more than meat, but a pig produces pork, bacon, ham and, of course, sausages.

This has huge advantages to the smallholder because it allows you to process your own products – and the more you do, the more value you add, so the more comfortable your profit margins. Better still, many of these 'added value' items use the shoulder and belly cuts, which can be difficult to shift with other large animals.

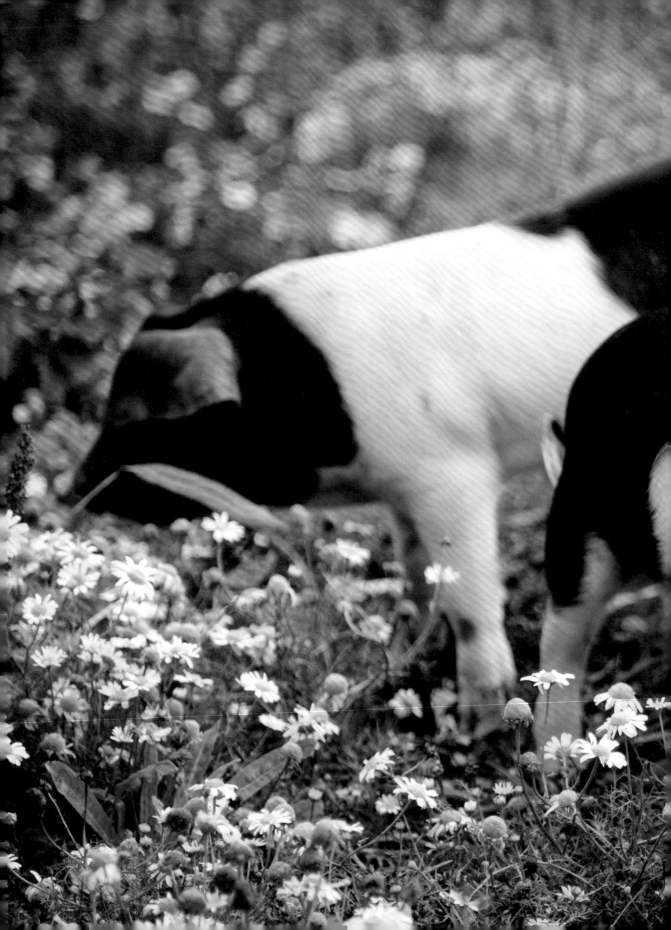

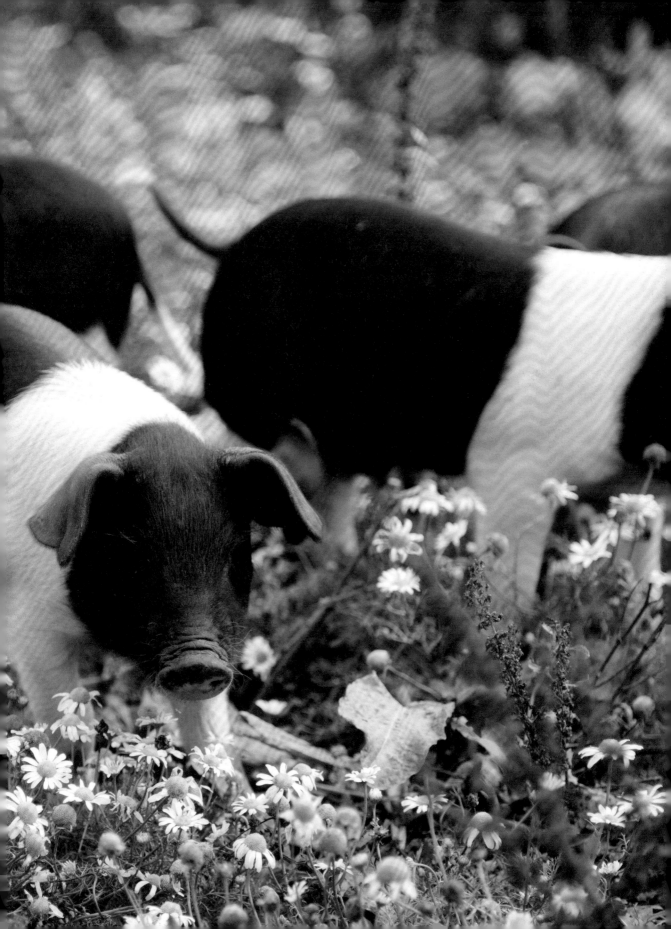

In my case it was the sausages that gave me the 'light bulb' moment. A good sausage needs a reasonable fat content if it is to stay moist and succulent, so the fattier parts of the animal are perfect for this. The big supermarkets usually sell these as an affordable simple product, but I realised that rather than this competition undercutting my margins, it actually gave me a real commercial opening. Cheap products use cheap ingredients – so mass-produced sausages use dried powdered flavourings and standardised rusk. There's nothing wrong with supplying profitable pork at a price people are willing to pay, and most commercial sausages are great value for what they are – an easily affordable family meal. However, I was convinced I could find discerning customers who would be prepared to pay more for a really excellent product. So by combining the superior texture and flavour of rare-breed pork with fresh herbs, real breadcrumbs and the best aromatic spices, I saw I could instantly lift what was already excellent meat up another two or three rungs.

Also I realised I could customise it further by thinking of original recipes that had a local feel. So where possible I researched old regional recipes and whenever I developed a new range I gave it a local name. We're based very firmly in East Anglia, so rather than simply producing 'Cumberland' or 'Lincolnshire' sausages when we are hundreds of miles away, I developed a similar herb-based variety called the 'St George'. We also sell the 'Ipswich Super Blue', which uses blue cheese and garlic and is a pun on the nickname of the local football team, and our plainest variety, the 'Classic Essex'. Similarly our leading bacon is called 'Colchester Forest' which harks back to the days when wild boar roamed in the local woods. All this allows me to charge three or four times as much for my products as the supermarkets ask for their economy versions.

Another hidden downside to rearing pigs for commercial gain is that the sheer range of products you can turn your hand to can lead to over-ambition. There are good reasons why salamis and Parma hams are so expensive – they have been matured for many months or years. This effectively locks away the return on your investment for up to two or three years. When I was in Spain recently I was shown a huge room full of Serrano hams which were maturing for two years before sale. I was told there was €2 million worth of ham in the one chamber – so, yes, curing a ham might turn a €20 cut into €200, but you are effectively loaning that money to your future customers rather than buying new stock or land. This also flags up another downside, in that now, almost without realising it, instead of competing against economy supermarket meat, you are competing against premium products created by Continental artisans. As a result, while I have found it relatively easy to carve a porcine niche in modern British retailing, I have reluctantly decided that creating my own version of a Continental ham is one step too far.

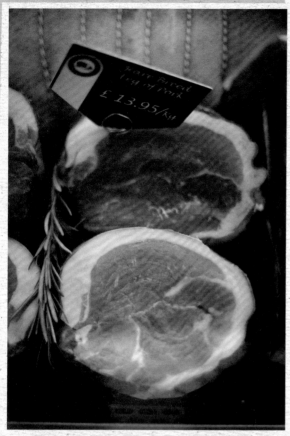

£ 13.95/kg

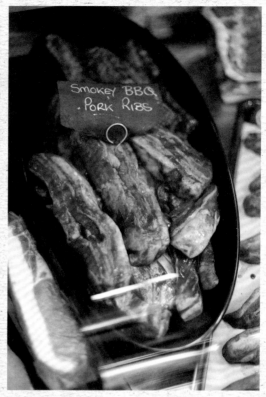

Smokey BBQ Pork Ribs

The Butc[her]

rm. To ensure
us rare breed

open pasture.
es!

here you are
ur food miles

us to survive

Our bacon is naturally dry cured her[e]
traditional, artisan methods. A combinatio[n]
is used to create a bacon of yesteryear
added preservatives. Our Smoked bacon is
and hickory chippings creating a superb [...]

Pig butchery diagram

- Head
- Cheeks/Jowel
- Spare Rib & Roast
- Blade
- Hand
- Loin
- Belly
- Trotter

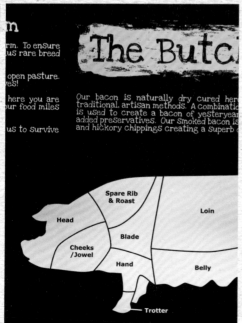

UNLIKE other BIG meat-producing ANIMALS, PIGS lend themselves to an unusually LARGE range of PRODUCTS.

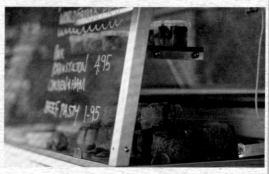

[...] 4.95

[...]HAM

BEEF PASTY 1.95

FOLLOWING THE PAPER TRAIL

Unfortunately pigs are probably the most legislated form of livestock you can keep, no matter how many or few you have. Some of this dates back to the days when many people had a pigsty in their garden. In towns and villages this could cause hygiene problems, so the earliest rules were intended to reduce legitimate problems. Then, during the Second World War, the government was worried about possible morale problems if heavily rationed townsfolk started to imagine their country cousins had access to plentiful pork and bacon. The biggest raft of legislation has been more recent, though; some of it stems from Europe, but most is related to animal welfare and control of highly infectious diseases such as foot and mouth.

This means that if you want to keep pigs you have to be capable of dealing with plenty of paperwork – and quite how much and how rigorously it is applied varies across the country and can also depend on the size of your herd. To start with you will need a holding number for your land and a herd number for your pigs. You get these from DEFRA or the devolved governments of Wales, Scotland and Northern Ireland. Before you fetch your pigs from the breeder or market, you will need a pig movement licence (which comes from your local council's trading standards office) and you will need another to take them to the abattoir. The pigs will also need a 'slap mark' – basically a tattoo with your holding number – which allows full traceability after death. On top of all this, you will probably be required to keep a medicines book, not to mention the extra layers of paperwork if you are in one of the growing range of organic and welfare certification schemes.

In the old days pigs were fed on food scraps and kitchen waste (I remember bins outside the school canteen labelled 'pig swill') but this could lead to disease problems, so first came strict rules about sterilising the food by cooking it all thoroughly. This was not enough to prevent the disastrous 2001 foot-and-mouth outbreak, however, so now it is illegal to feed them any waste food and you have to sign all sorts of declarations to this effect when you take them to the abattoir.

All this can sound terrifying to the beginner, but in fact it's much easier than it first appears. To start with you do almost everything yourself, so your trading standards office will give you a pile of blank movement licences which you simply fill out when you take your pigs anywhere. The 'slap mark' tattoo is no more than a stick with a pad on the end bearing a series of pins shaped in the appropriate letters and numbers. You push this into an ink pad and then whack it onto your pig to leave an indelible number in their skin (hence the name 'slap mark'). They jump a little when you do this, but within moments they will be happily eating away and will have forgotten all about it.

All this information is easily available online from the Department of Environment, Food and Rural Affairs or the appropriate regionally devolved government. Trading Standards officers are generally very helpful too, particularly if you only have a few animals. As always, it is a really good idea to talk to another pig keeper and, better still, the appropriate rare breed society.

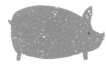

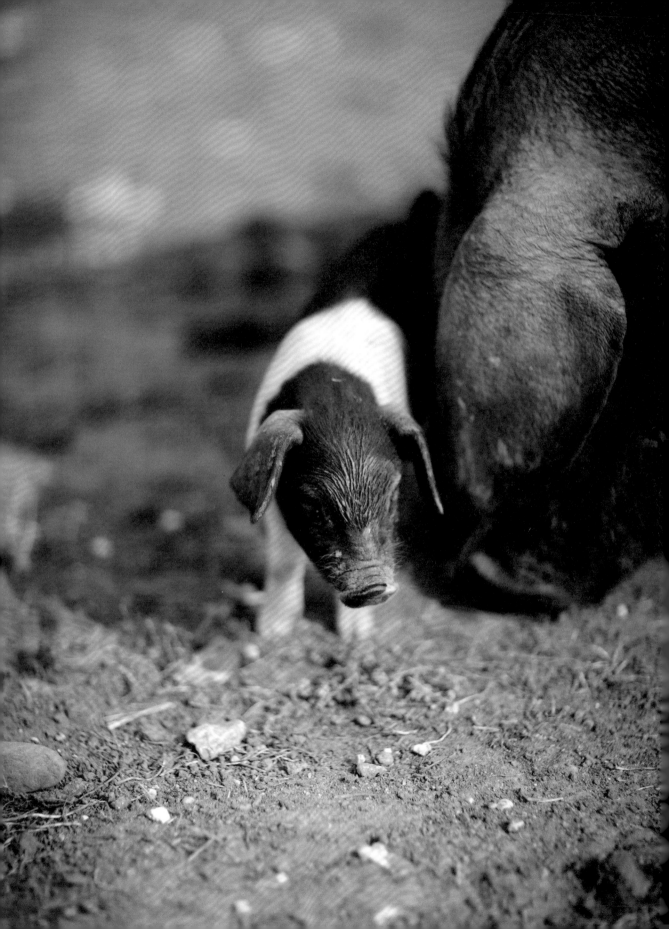

Cattle

In theory cattle are an attractive option for those with a few acres. They produce a lot of premium meat and are generally fairly trouble-free – at least they are if you opt for the older, tougher breeds like the Dexter, Welsh black or Highland. If you go for a traditional, dual-purpose breed you could even milk them to produce your own farmhouse cheese or yoghurt. Certainly they have long been the backbone of British lowland agriculture as an animal that provides multiple products; cows provide almost all the milk we consume, and it can be readily turned into butter, cheese, cream and yoghurt. The meat, too, is one of our favourite staples and most cuts command a good price. Even the bones can be rendered down to provide stock, gelatine or glue, while the skin tans readily to provide leather.

They need a lot of space, however. A cow and calf might be able to find all the food they need on 0.2 hectare (a half acre) in summer, but they either need a lot more ground or bought-in fodder in winter. This is particularly true for dairy cattle. Milk is full of protein and to get good yields the cow will need plenty of rich grazing in summer and concentrates in the form of hay in winter. Even a small cow will need something like an acre of grass if kept outside all year round (even more on poor ground). The hardier species such as Highlands have no need of shelter in winter, but most of the others do much better with indoor protection.

As with sheep, post foot and mouth cattle involve a lot of paperwork and record keeping. Each has to be individually tagged, its movements carefully logged and you will need to keep a medicines book too.

Problems

Their hooves, combined with their weight, mean that cattle will soon make a mess of wet ground. They are also slow growing, so unless you are thinking of producing veal, they will take at least 18 months to reach killing weight. In fact, 30 months (the oldest a beef animal can be killed, thanks to post-BSE regulations) is generally better. Ironically, however, when they are this big the small producer can face a problem of too much meat. Some beef breeds can weigh over a tonne – far too much for a family to store and consumer easily.

Likewise, a dairy cow could produce four or five litres of milk a day – again, far too much for one family yet far too little for the wholesalers. The answer, of course, is to process it into cheese, butter and yoghurt for sale, but while four to five litres of milk is too much for a family to consume, many cheese recipes require larger amounts of milk to work. Manufacturing dairy products also requires specialist equipment and scrupulous cleanliness, however

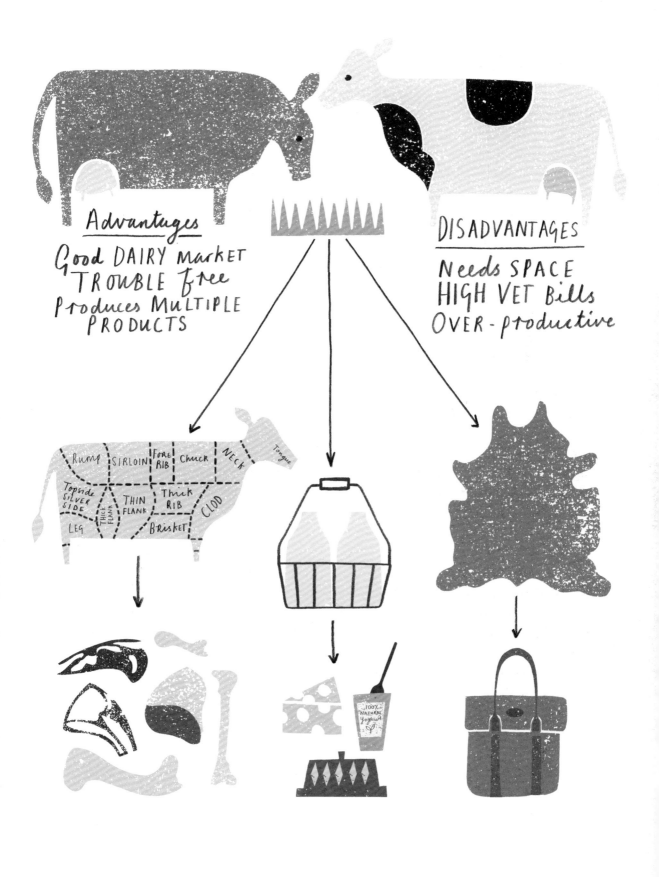

Advantages
Good DAIRY market
TROUBLE free
Produces MULTIPLE
PRODUCTS

DISADVANTAGES
Needs SPACE
HIGH VET Bills
OVER-productive

Rump SIRLOIN FORE RIB Chuck NECK Tongue
Topside SILVER SIDE THIN FLANK Thick RIB CLOD
THICK FLANK LEG Brisket

100% NATURAL Yoghurt

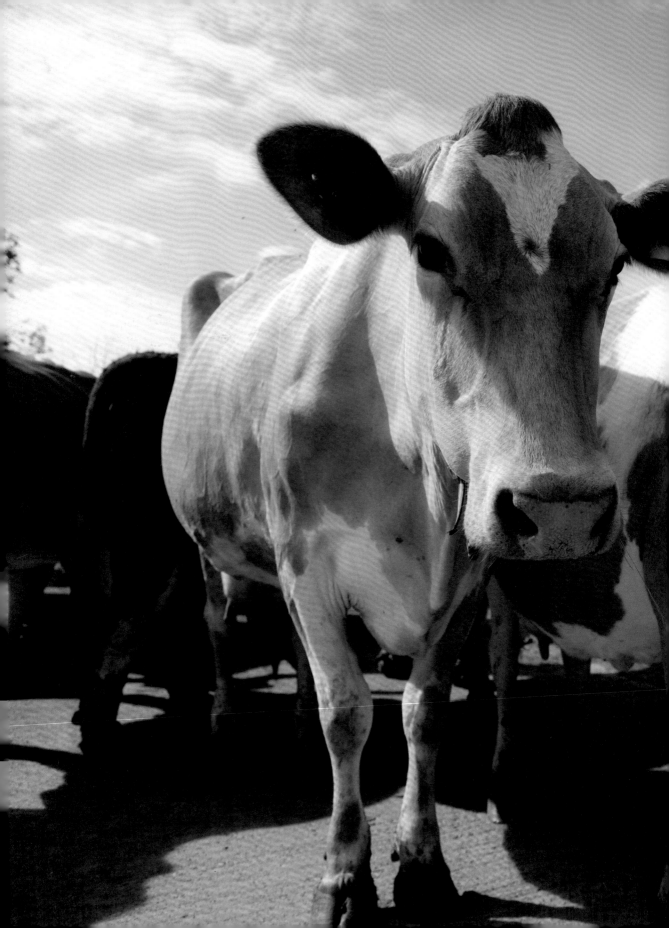

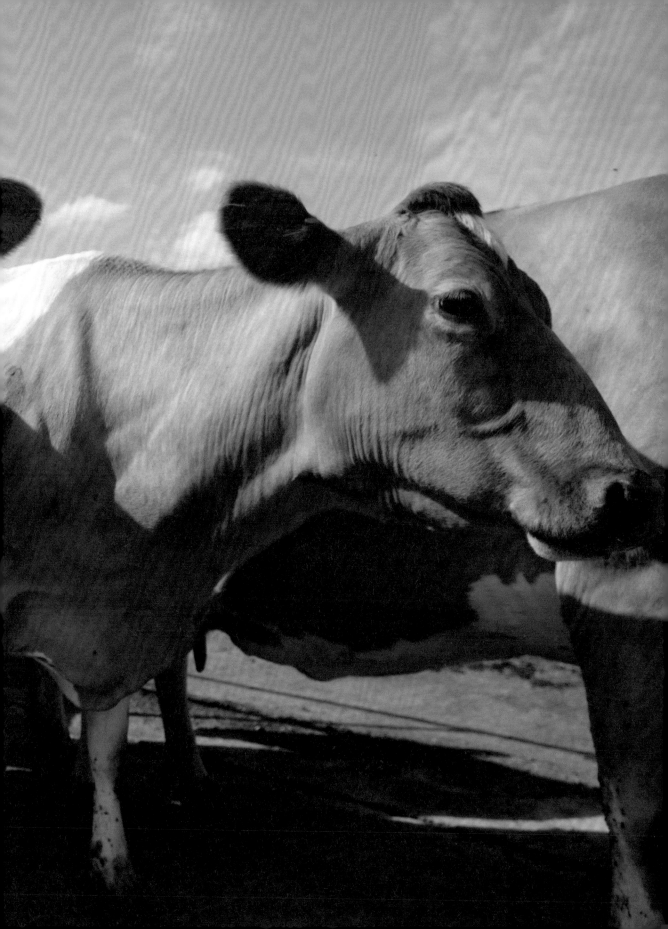

(which can be difficult on a working farm), and you will get regular health inspections. It is also a huge ongoing commitment.

Most cattle are generally healthy, but when one does fall ill, their size means this involves a home visit from the vet, which means a substantial bill. As a result, most farmers keep a medicine cabinet of routine drugs to inject into the animals themselves and are also capable of minor birthing interventions. Farming cattle is not for the squeamish.

Breeds

Hundreds of cattle strains have been developed all over the world, each designed to fit various local needs. As with all livestock, before buying animals check what neighbours are doing and seek advice, but because this is a competitive market choosing an unusual breed might give you the edge you need.

Charolais: A huge cream beef breed that originated in Burgundy but is now found all over the world. In Britain it is often crossed with native breeds like the Hereford and Aberdeen Angus to produce animals with the right muscle-to-fat ratio loved by butchers.

Hereford: A great beef animal which was exported all over the world during the nineteenth century.

Holstein-Friesian: The classic black-and-white dual-purpose breed that underpins most of Britain's modern dairy products yet also produces acceptable meat. Recently, however, animal rights activists have highlighted welfare problems linked to the huge size and weight of the udders, which can produce over 2,800 litres of milk every year.

Dexter: If you are going to keep cattle, then arguably this is the perfect smallholder's breed. Although slow-growing and only reaching half to a third of the size of a Hereford or Friesian, these cows produce good-quality milk, a decent carcass and can even be used as draft oxen.

Highland: This shaggy horned creature is extremely hardy, which makes it ideal for colder conditions and poorer land. It also produces a good carcass. Its wonderful appearance and docile temperament mean it is ideal for set-ups with a visitor element.

Selling your produce

If you do decide to produce dairy products, make sure you have a decent product so that the 'artisan' component will do most of your marketing for you. You are still in competition with the mass-produced output of Britain's big creameries and Continental imports, however, so it will be vital to stress that your cheese is handmade and local.

Beef is more difficult to sell commercially, but not impossible. An unusual traditional breed and organic or welfare-scheme registration are good starting points. One major problem is the sheer volume of meat and variety of cuts you will have to shift from even one

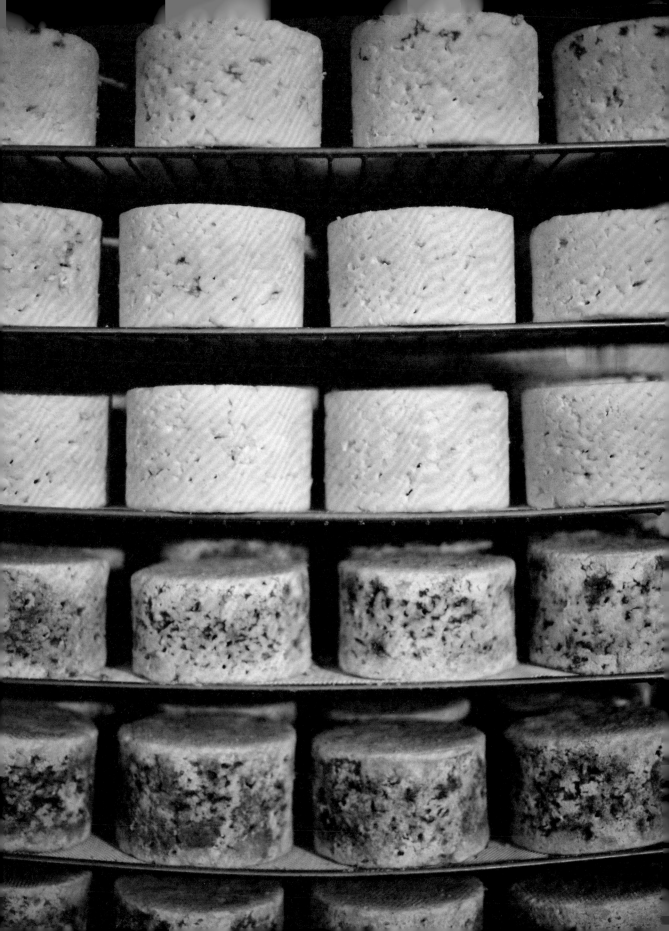

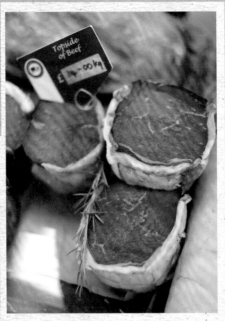

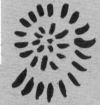

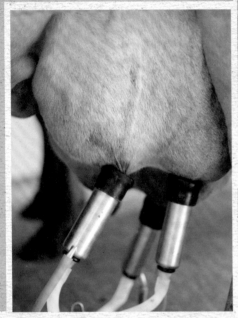

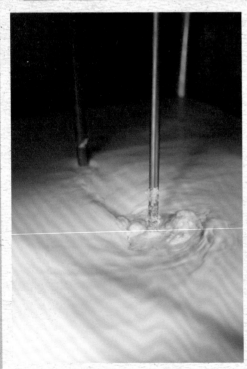

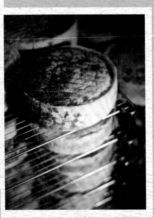

COWS not only PROVIDE one of OUR STAPLE Meats, but almost all the MILk we BRITISH Consume, Which can BE TURNED into BUTTER, CHEESE, CREAM and Yoghurt

animal. The simplest solution is to sell the whole carcass to a traditional butcher who will sell your animal to his customers labelled with your farm name and the rearing details.

Although this is much the simplest way of selling, it does give the butcher an important slice of added value, so if you sell the meat directly yourself you can cash in on this and add other elements to the product. One of the most important ways of doing this is to mature the meat properly for up to a month. This has to happen in controlled conditions, but when done correctly it allows harmless micro-organisms to start the decay process, sweetening and tenderising the meat so that it slowly turns from bright red to brown. Unfortunately too many consumers associate the vibrant red of very fresh meat with quality, so although well-matured beef wins hands down in taste tests, it is vital to explain the process to customers (ideally backed up with samples to prove the point).

About half an animal can be butchered into the prime steaks and roasting joints, but most customers don't have the time or culinary knowledge to deal with the tougher cuts (for example, shin and skirt). Providing printed and online cooking tips and recipes will reduce the problem, but you will still be left with a lot of meat. This is where processing the meat into sausages, ready-meals and burgers is not only an option, but probably essential. Once again you will have to aim for the highest quality and stress the uniqueness of the products.

One sideline of rearing cattle can be its skin. A cow produces a very large and potentially valuable skin which can be turned into leather. Most abattoirs take this in part-payment for slaughtering, but you can ask for it back if you want to process this at home. However, it is a messy and smelly job and can easily go wrong. That said, some producers are now organically tanning hides using traditional methods and creating a luxury product such as a whole-hide hair-on rug.

Over the centuries man has harnessed the qualities of a huge range of livestock. There is no reason why that should not continue today. So unless you are a vegan or you live in a tiny basement flat, there is actually every possibility that you can keep at least some living creature as part of your home-production process. At the smallest end of the scale this might be bees to help pollinate your crops, while if you have a scrap of garden, a few bantams will recycle your kitchen waste into more eggs than you can eat. Given a bigger garden of small paddock, pigs will help prepare the ground while producing the most succulent organic pork, bacon and sausages you can imagine. Most ambitious of all, perhaps, would be a milking goat or cow which would allow you to produce delicious farmhouse cheeses and yoghurts flavoured with your own soft fruit. They are, after all, part of the natural cycle of life and your plot will be enriched with their presence – in every sense.

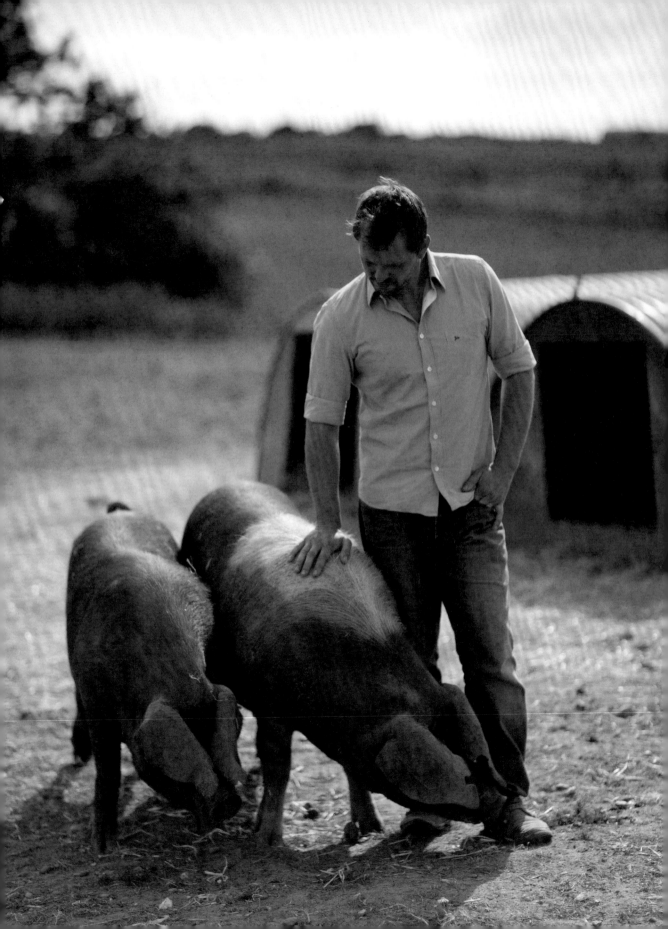

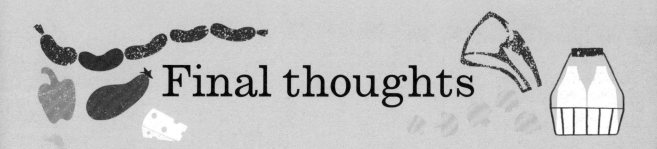

Final thoughts

Anyone who loves food has to count themselves lucky to be alive today. Thanks to the culinary revolution over the past 30 years or so, we now have access to a staggering array of high-quality British ingredients which would have been far beyond our reach in the dark days of post-war austerity.

Much of the credit must go to the great cookery writers such as Elizabeth David and Jane Grigson. Fantastic chefs such as Raymond Blanc, the Roux brothers and Antonio Carluccio have played their part too, first by building up award-winning restaurants which set the standard for others, then later by being publicists for great cooking on television and in print.

Then, of course, there are the producers themselves – people who are passionate about a particular product and pump all their time and effort into creating something of which they are truly proud. But, however great the produce (and many really are the best in the world), ultimately the credit has to go to the consumers who have dared to experiment when eating out and later back in their own kitchens. We farmers can only rear and grow great food if the public is prepared to buy it.

A lot of people think my farming business only took off because of my TV work. Actually that's just not true. For a start, while I really enjoyed the shows, filming was a huge distraction from the work that had to be done. I was standing in front of cameras doing take after take because the lighting or sound weren't quite right when I could have been making sausages or putting up a new fence. Certainly, I got a lot of free publicity, and that did draw in the crowds, but the problem is it's quite ephemeral. You have to take on more staff to cater for the rush, but a few weeks later the crowds have gone and you've still got a whopping wage bill. In the end you have to lay people off, and that's really gut-wrenching.

Where TV did help, however, was by introducing me to a huge number of really imaginative smallholders and gardeners

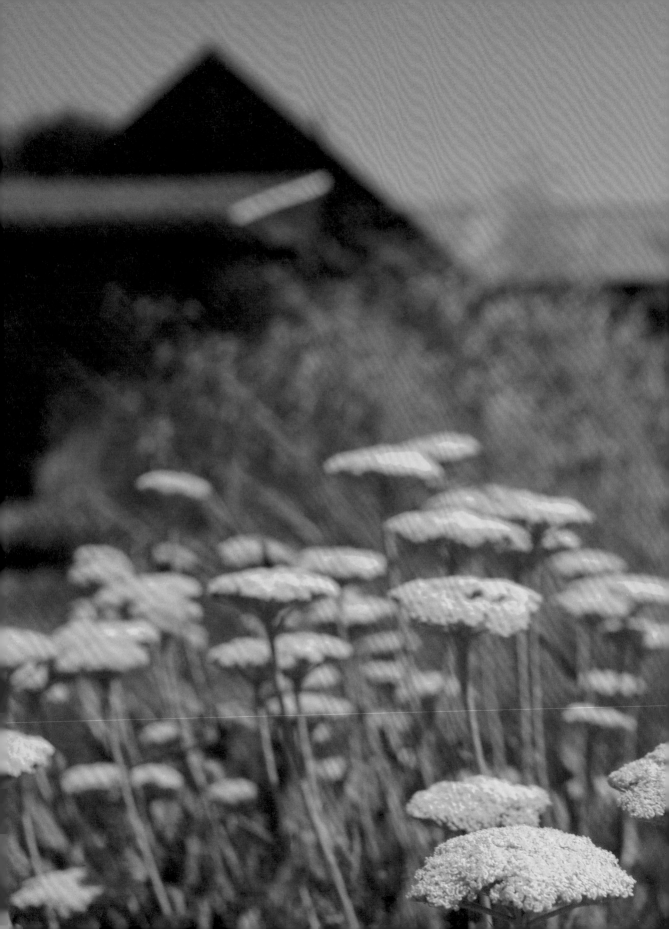

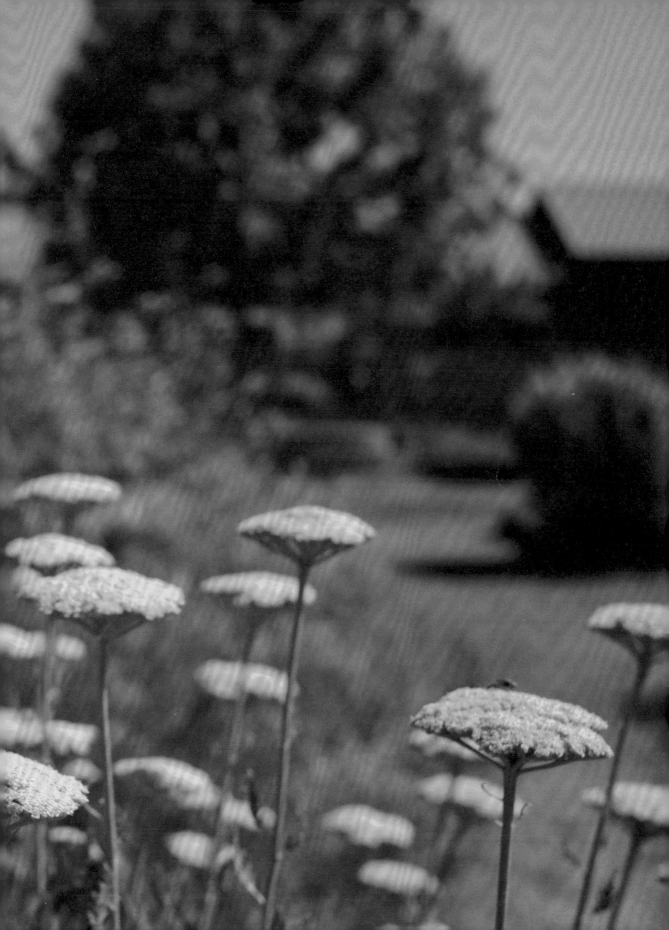

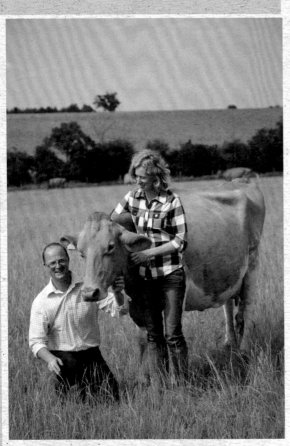

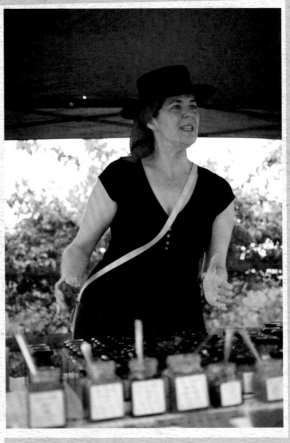

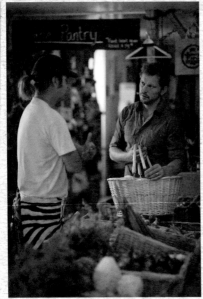

I TAKE MY HAT off to the PIGS, other Farmers and PRODUCERS, but most of all to the GREAT BRITISH PUBLIC who Buy my produce and make it all Possible.

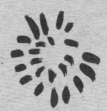

across the country. There are hundreds of people out there who are completely dedicated to growing, rearing and making high-quality produce. Talking to them has been fascinating and a huge source of inspiration.

One idea is to go back to the ancient pig-farming technique of 'pannage', by which a village would drive its pigs into the woods in autumn to fatten them up on acorns. The first time I tried this I put too many into too small a wood and they killed some of the smaller trees, but the idea is still basically a sound one. I am now planning to buy a few old parachutes and I will spread these out beneath the oaks in the autumn to catch the falling acorns, which we will then store and feed to the pigs as part of their balanced diet.

The music festival is another exciting development. This event brings thousands of visitors to the farm for a weekend in early September. And there's a twist: on one stage we have great bands playing while on the second we have cookery demonstrations and talks – in other words, we're combining two of my favourite pastimes and attracting a new group of customers.

My latest project has been to convert one of the old barns into a restaurant where, as well as the usual fare, we have a 'head to tail' menu. This makes a virtue out of using up every bit of the pig. So we make the hearts and livers into faggots; the fattier slivers go into that gorgeous French potted meat 'rillettes'. We also have crispy pigs' ears and tails, turn the heads into brawn, and bone out and stuff

the trotters. It really is a case of using everything but the 'oink'.

Looking ahead, I can't help noticing that we've got another derelict barn. I'd love to convert this too. We'd let it out on a peppercorn rent to someone to set up a children's playgroup. I like the idea of there being kids around here, but even better it will mean that their parents are coming to drop them off and pick them up twice a day, and as they do so, they drive past our shop. It might sound a bit cynical, but it's not – no one is going to give them the hard sell, but as a producer you have to think laterally – how can you increase the number of potential customers?

Becoming a pig farmer has been hugely rewarding and great fun. I love my animals, and spending time with them has been a fantastic privilege. I've also enjoyed turning the meat into produce which I think is as good as any in the world. It has also been just the start of a wonderful learning process. I am still learning and experimenting today: I hope I will still be open to new ideas when I am in my dotage. So I take my hat off to the pigs, other farmers and producers, but most of all to the great British public who buy my produce and make it all possible.

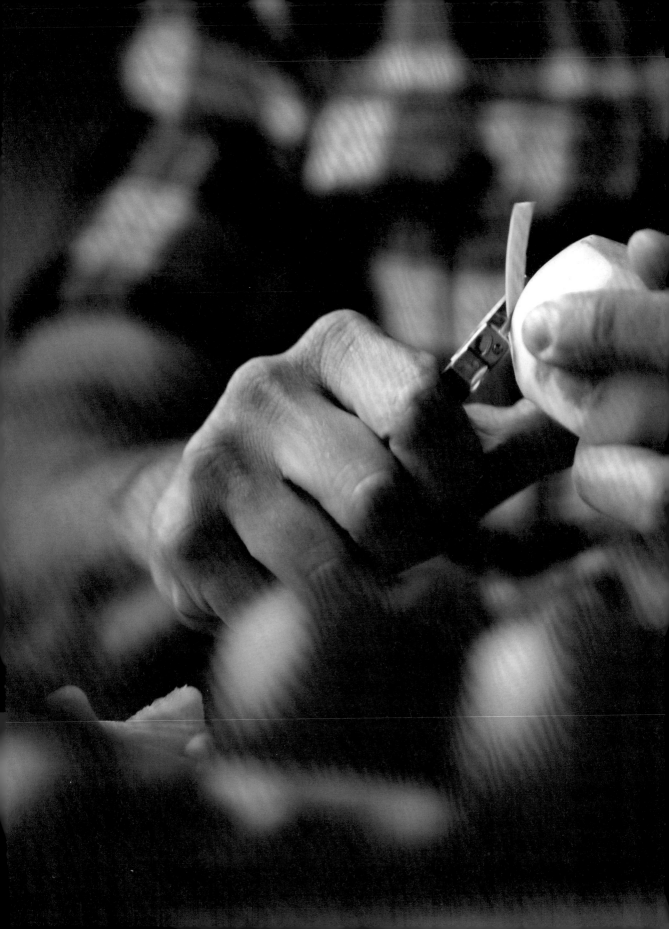

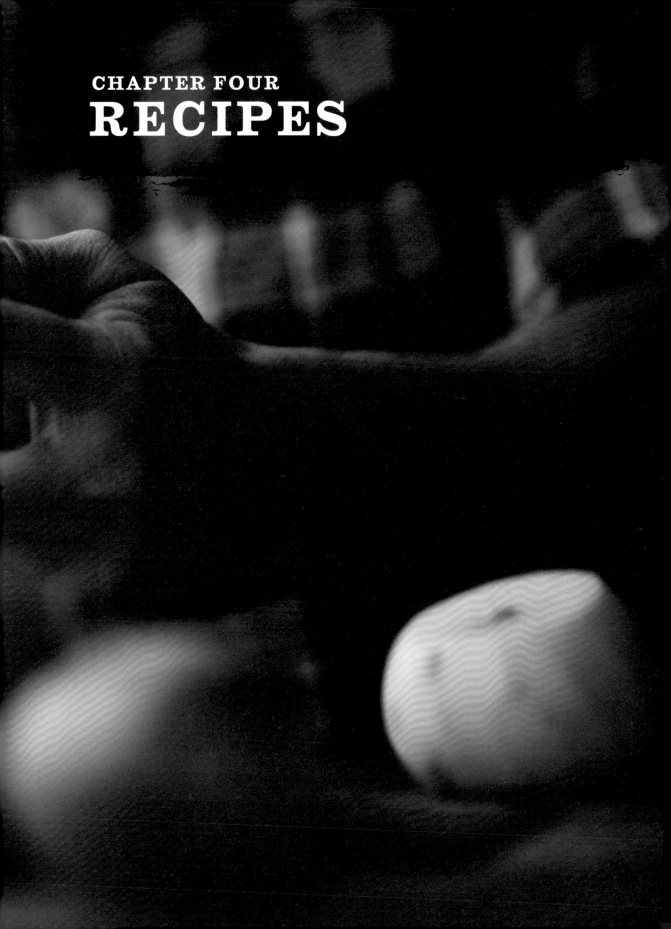

CHAPTER FOUR
RECIPES

APPLE AND ROSEMARY JELLY

Most autumns there is an abundance of apples it seems a pity to waste. Many will keep well deep into winter if picked carefully from the tree, wrapped in a twist of paper, popped into a shallow box with a small gap between each fruit and stored in a cool dry cellar or garage. This doesn't work for windfalls, though, and crab apples and 'wildings' (the descendants of apple cores that are locally abundant along towpaths and hedges) are generally too bitter for consumption. All apples are high in pectin, however, which makes them ideal for jellies. On their own apples tend to be a little bland, but they make a great 'base' for flavoured jellies, harnessing the transient aromatic tastes of summer for use throughout the year.

Of course, the most familiar form of using a herb this way is the traditional mint jelly. There is nothing wrong with this, but to my mind it is a little dull – particularly after mixing with vinegar to make mint sauce. This recipe uses rosemary and, like the mint version, it makes a great condiment to serve with lamb dishes.

You can use the same basic method to create a range of aromatic accompaniments and, thanks to the sugar, they also make a fantastic glaze for roast meats such as venison and pork. Thus the addition of oregano, chilli, rowan berries or even lavender can give an unusual flavour to a familiar dish.

MAKES 2 JARS
2kg tart apples (for example cookers, crabs or wildings)
Cold water to cover
1.5kg preserving sugar
Big bunch rosemary
   (or your preferred herb)

1 Chop the apples roughly and put them in a large pan with almost all the rosemary. Pour in enough water to cover most of the apples, cover, mash occasionally and simmer until everything is soft (about 45 minutes).

2 Pour the fruit and herb mix into a jelly bag and leave to drip for a couple of hours, speeding up the final stages by squeezing the juices out with your hands. Measure the juice and add 500g of sugar for every 500ml of liquid. Return to the boil and simmer for 15 minutes – then pour into sterilised jars, carefully adding a sprig of rosemary (or whatever herb, spice or flavouring you are using), to the centre as decoration.

3 It should keep for up to two years – although ideally you should store jars in a fridge once opened.

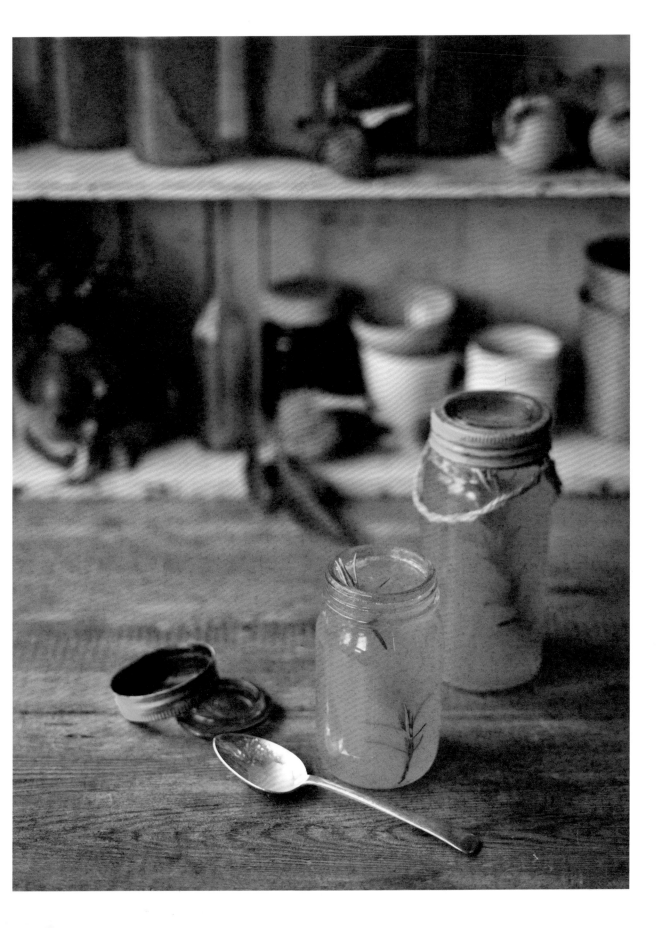

JAM

We think of jam as no more than a sweet addition to toast and butter, but in the past it was an important way of storing vitamin C for the long winter months. Although the principles of using sugar to chemically preserve foods were first discovered in the Middle Ages, the sweetener's high price meant it was beyond the reach of most pockets. This changed during the course of the eighteenth century, when the slave trade saw the establishment of vast plantations in the Americas. As a result its price tumbled and soon most British kitchens had a miniature production line every autumn.

The basic principles are simple: the high concentration of sugars effectively locks up all the water at the microscopic level, making life impossible for the bacteria and fungi which would otherwise quickly spoil the individual ingredients.

The other issue with jam making, however, is the need for the natural setting agent: pectin. This occurs naturally in fruit such as apples, although some soft fruit such as strawberries can struggle to produce enough to gel. The answer is to use a mixture of ingredients, add jam-making sugar (which contains pectin) or add it yourself.

If you are making jam, rather than simply making a 'straight' one-fruit variety, it is a good idea to use a mixture of fruits to create something which simply isn't available in the shops. This recipe works well and gives the basic method, but once you have succeeded with a couple of batches you should start to experiment with quantities and ingredients to create something which is genuinely your own.

JUMBLE FRUIT JAM
MAKES 1.5KG
1.2kg mixed fruit (e.g. strawberries, currants, possibly supplemented with hedgerow fruit such as black- and bilberries)
Juice and zest of 1 orange
Juice and zest of 1 lemon
Juice and zest of 1 lime
1kg preserving sugar
125ml water

1 Put the cleaned fruit into a pan with the other ingredients. Leave to marinate for 1–2 hours, letting the juices seep out. Transfer to a pan and gently heat, stirring occasionally as the juices soften the fruit and dissolve the sugar. Raise the heat to boil for about 10 minutes until it reaches setting point (to determine this, put a dab on a chilled plate – after a minute draw the back of a spoon across the dollop – if the surface wrinkles, it's there). Do not overcook, because ideally you want your jam to have texture as well as a great taste. If things go too far, you can always pour it through a jelly bag, squeezing out the excess juices to create a lovely thick condiment.

2 Pour into sterilised jars and seal tightly – it should keep for well over a year.

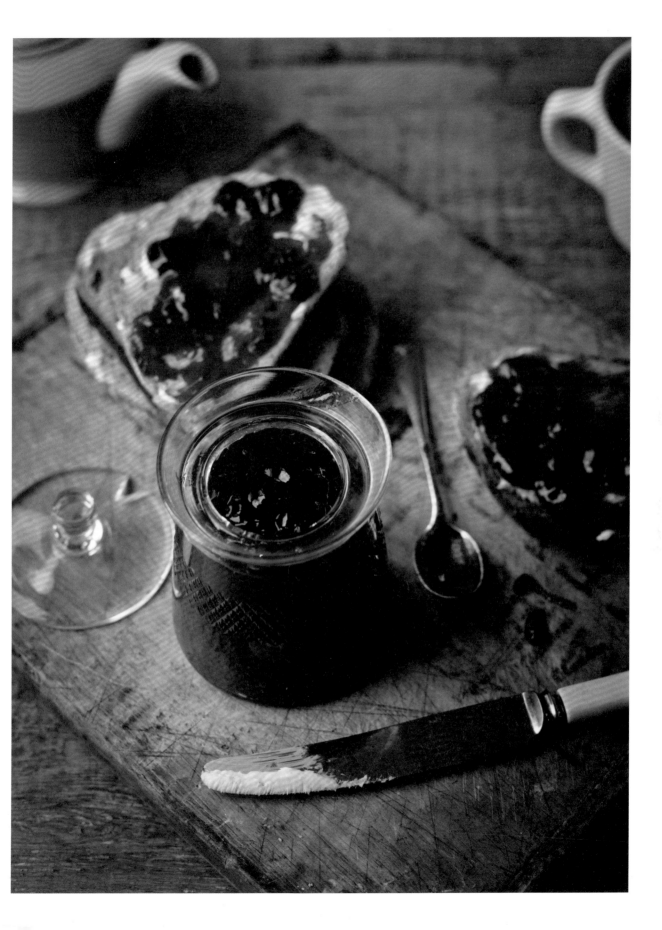

SMOKED CHILLI OIL

This is incredibly easy to make and produces a fantastic oil which is great as either an ingredient or a condiment. Smoking the chillies is much simpler than you might imagine. You can use a special smoker (see pp. 155–6), but a conventional 'kettle' barbecue is just as good and much cheaper and simpler for most people. The important thing is to keep the temperature down – you want to smoke the fruit, not toast it to a crisp. One way of doing this is to have a normal barbecue with friends and then, as the last coals glow gently among the ash, put on handfuls of hardwood shavings (you can buy these loose or as pellets from the internet, or ask a local joiner for his waste shavings). The other consideration is what strength you want – this is obviously going to depend most on the type of chilli, but there will always be a fair amount of trial and error. If you end up with something which is far too fiery, make another batch using sweet peppers instead and then blend the two batches.

250g chillies
2 bulbs garlic (whole)
5 bay leaves
2 litres sunflower oil
30 green peppercorns

1 Put the chillies and garlic as high above the heat as possible and cover. Check regularly to ensure the fire is still producing smoke and the heat hasn't crept up too high. Cooking times vary on the intensity and temperature of the smoke, and even climatic conditions, so it is impossible to give precise times. The longer you smoke, the more powerful the flavour: 2–3 hours is probably about right.

2 Put the chillies, garlic and bay leaves into a food processor. Pour in a little oil and whizz to a rough paste. Tip into the biggest jar you can find (old-fashioned sweetie jars are ideal, or buy an equivalent storage jar). Add the peppercorns, then wash out the processor bowl with oil to get the last of the chilli and garlic paste. Top up with the rest of the oil, tightly seal the jar and put in a dark cupboard for a couple of months (test it for outline flavour after a day or so).

3 Divide the oil amongst smaller bottles or jars. You can strain or even filter it, but it will be cloudy and it looks good with a sediment layer at the bottom. If you are giving it as a present or selling it, dress it up by using attractive bottles and waxing the corks. Once opened it will keep for several months – although it is so delicious it rarely lasts that long.

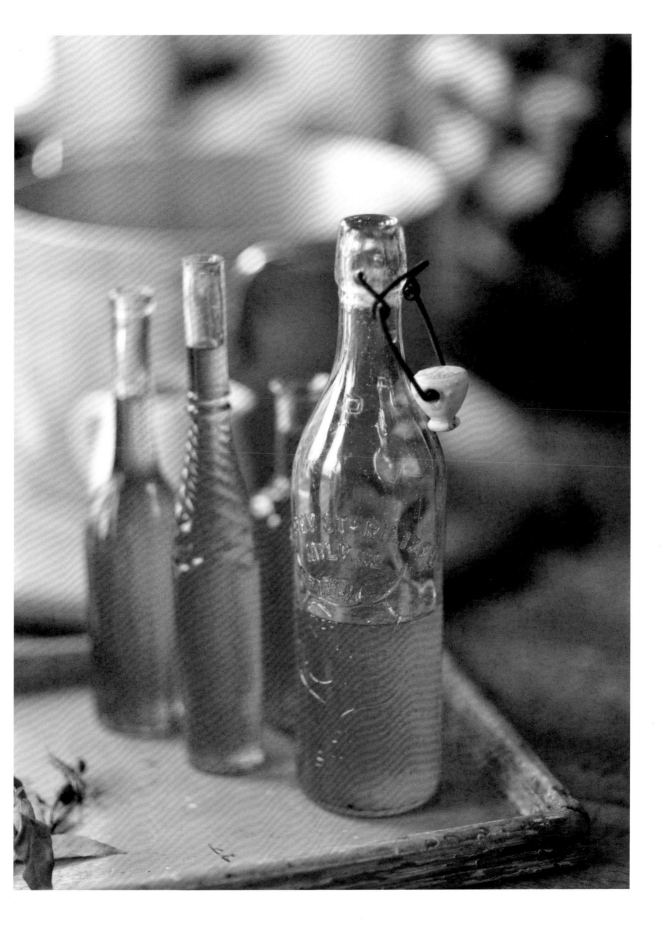

CHUTNEY

The English word comes from the Hindi '*catni*', a thick – usually aromatic or spicy – relish served alongside a main dish. There are hundreds, perhaps thousands, of regional variations on the sub-continent, varying from delicately scented coriander and mint dishes to fiery chilli-based condiments. Chutneys were introduced to Britain by soldiers and civil servants returning from the Raj and, as with so many Indian dishes, chutneys have become heavily adapted in the process.

As well as being an interesting addition to all sorts of dishes, meats and cheeses, chutneys are a great way of preserving the annual summer glut of vegetables and fruit. For example, in a bumper year you might want to turn spare plums or damsons into a spicy accompaniment for meat or a soft cheese like Camembert.

The basic chemistry behind a chutney relies on the combination of sweet and sour natural preservatives, The first is generally sugar, the second citrus juice or vinegar. These are then perked up with various spices or herbs. It goes without saying, though, that the better the sugar and vinegar you use, the better the end result – so don't skimp on these. When you have mastered the techniques, you can invent your own recipes, juggling the ingredients and quantities of spices to create a range of 'signature' condiments. This basic recipe, however, harnesses the almost inevitable embarrassment of overgrown late-summer courgettes.

MARROW CHUTNEY
2 onions, chopped
500g diced marrow
500g chopped tomatoes
300ml cider vinegar
2 Bramley apples,
   peeled and diced
250g muscovado sugar
6 garlic cloves
5cm cinnamon stick
5cm knob of root ginger,
   grated
1–4 chopped chillies
   (according to taste)
6 cloves
6 cardamom pods
1 tbsp coriander seeds
1 tbsp mustard seeds

1 Put all the ingredients into a large saucepan, bring slowly to bubbling point and then simmer gently for 2 hours until thick, brown and shiny. Pour into sterilised jars and seal tightly. Leave to mature for at least three weeks.

2 The chutney should keep in the sealed jars for at least a year, but store in a fridge once opened and they will last comfortably for several weeks.

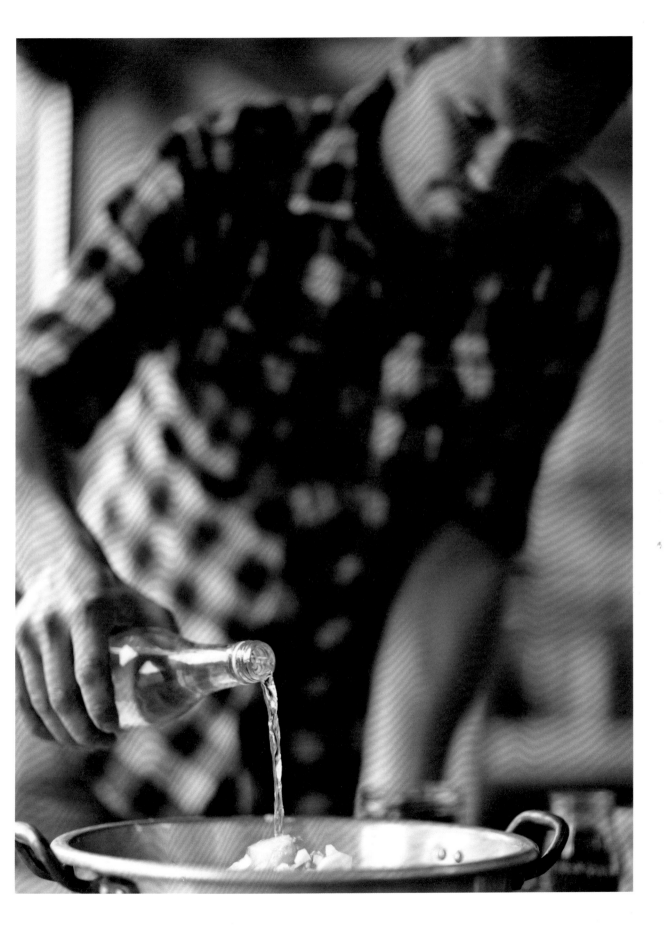

GAME PÂTÉ

Pâté is a simple and delicious way of transforming inexpensive or potentially tough cuts of meat into a premium product. This recipe is particularly good for turning the abundance of autumnal game into a tasty dish which even fussy kids will love. The secret of a good pâté is having a relatively high fat content, but game is almost devoid of this (which is why it is so healthy). As a result it requires a lot of added fat to stay moist. This comes from bacon, belly pork and back fat (while chicken liver pâté usually gets this from butter and cream). As a rough rule of thumb you need roughly two-parts fatty meat to one-part game, plus more fat to line the dish. This recipe is based very loosely on one by Elizabeth David, but here the flavour is intensified by using venison instead of veal, more duck, pheasant or rabbit, and by adding more juniper berries (which pump up the gamey taste). If you want an even stronger flavour, you could add a tablespoon of brined green peppercorns.

1 wild duck
1 pheasant or rabbit
150ml dry white wine
750g pork back fat
1kg pork belly
  (coarsely minced)
1kg stewing venison
  (coarsely minced)
3 large garlic cloves
4–5 sprigs of thyme
100ml cognac or calvados
20 juniper berries
10 black peppercorns
½ tsp cayenne pepper
2 bay leaves

1 Put the duck and pheasant or rabbit in a pan and roast in a moderate oven for 20 minutes. The meat should be pink and moist. Remove the skin from the duck and pare off as much meat as you can from the bones. Return the bones to the hot oven for a few minutes to brown, then put them into a pan and boil vigorously (deglaze the roasting pan with a splash of wine and water to catch the cooking juices).

2 Coarsely chop the cooked meat and 100g of the back fat and add to the minced pork and venison. Crush the garlic and strip the thyme leaves from the stalks and add to the meat. Pour in the white wine and cognac, season lightly with salt and pepper and marinate in the fridge overnight.

3 Meanwhile, put the browned bones, duck skin and any trimmings in a pan with the juniper berries, peppercorns, cayenne and bay leaves. Cover with water and boil vigorously until reduced to about 2 tablespoons. Strain, add to the meat and mix well.

4 Turn the meat into a terrine and cover the top with a lattice of fine strips of pork fat. Cover with foil and stand in a baking tin containing water. Cook in a low oven for 2 hours, removing the foil for the last 15 minutes to brown.

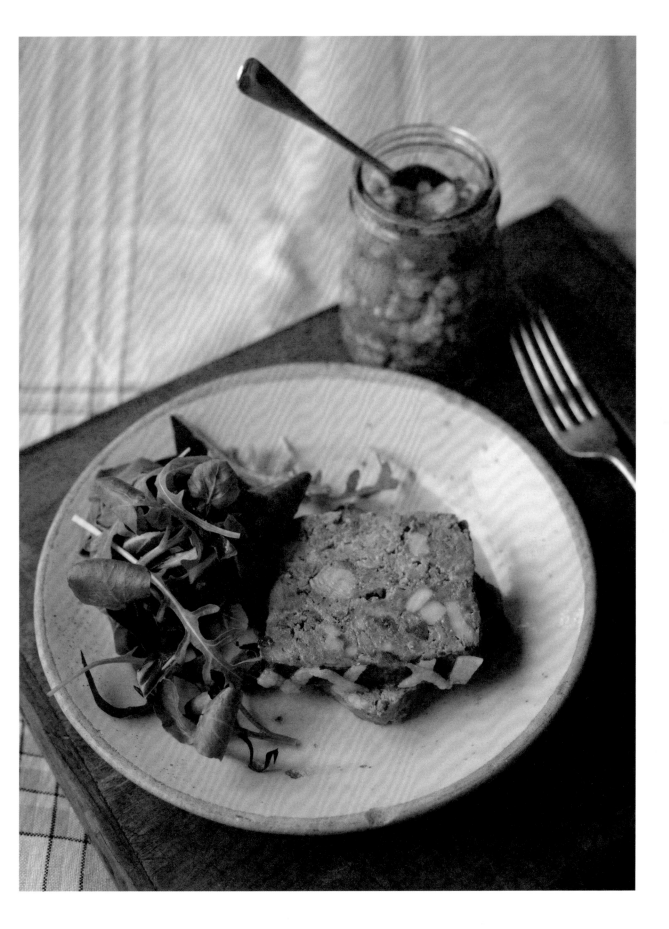

SUCCULENT SAUSAGES

For years the sausage was the perfect way to use up the fattier cuts of meat. Unfortunately, it is also a great way to get rid of all sorts of otherwise unsaleable matter, and so as a result they started to get a tarnished reputation. This is such a pity because a good sausage makes a wonderfully simple meal, and if you start to play around creating your own recipes the possibilities are literally endless.

Making sausages is definitely an art, although not a particularly difficult one to master (you don't need to go on a course to learn the basic secrets, but if you can persuade your butcher to let you watch him making a batch this will be invaluable). Sausages can be made with just a funnel and a wooden spoon, but it is much simpler to use a food processor with a mincer and sausage-making attachment. These are still being manufactured, but you may need to shop around on the internet or in specialist cookery shops. If you ask your nearest traditional butcher nicely, you can normally persuade him to sell you some casings (which are generally cleaned sheep intestines), but if this doesn't work there are mail-order suppliers.

In these health-obsessed days it might be tempting to cut down on the fat content, but this is a mistake – a decent amount of back or belly fat is vital for texture and flavour. Something like one-part fat to two-parts lean is roughly right. I try to include as much meat as possible in my sausages: at least 85 per cent and possibly up to 95 per cent (this includes fat). Obviously a small proportion of the remainder will be taken up by the flavourings, but the other vital ingredient is some sort of binding – if you make a pure meat sausage you will find a lot of the fat drains out into the pan and the texture becomes very dense – chewy even. The binding helps to hold in the fat and flavours, creating a more succulent and tasty end result. Traditionally butchers used stale bread from the local bakery or some sort of flour such as oatmeal, but today most sausages contain a commercial rusk which, again, you can usually get from a friendly butcher. The texture is also hugely affected by how finely the meat is minced. Personally I think a coarser mincing plate is best, although sometimes I run it twice through the machine to break it up a little more. In some areas, such as the Midlands, they like a finer texture and mince it several times with the finest cutting plate.

There are, of course, an infinite variety of recipes and it is great fun inventing your own. I think it is generally best to keep it fairly simple, though. There is a very good reason why the most popular sausages, like Lincolnshire (sage) or Cumberland (black pepper), are based around one or two dominant flavourings. So, once you've mastered the basic sausage, experiment with freshly chopped chillies, herbs; garlic or spices such as nutmeg, chilli, cumin and coriander.

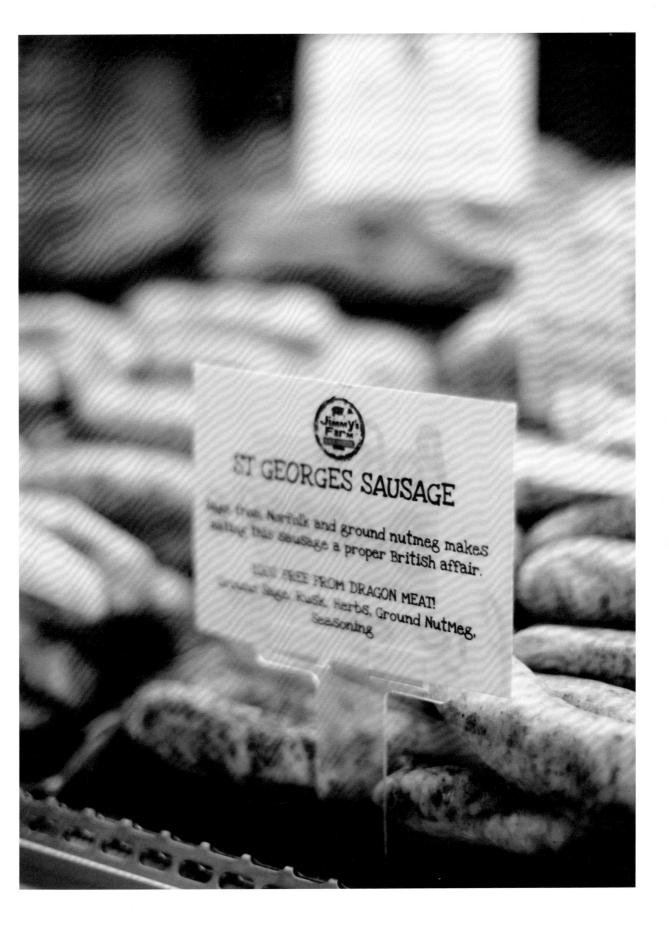

ST GEORGES SAUSAGE

Sage from Norfolk and ground nutmeg makes eating this sausage a proper British affair.

100% FREE FROM DRAGON MEAT!

Ground Sage, Rusk, Herbs, Ground Nutmeg, Seasoning

SAUSAGE RECIPE

**MAKES 15–20 LARGE
SAUSAGES**
500g minced pork
**500g pork diced into 5mm
  cubes**
**50g toasted breadcrumbs
  (about 2–3 slices of bread)**
2 tsp sea salt
2 tsp cracked black pepper
**Sausage skins (available from
  all good butchers)**

1 Place the minced and diced pork in a large bowl
with the breadcrumbs, salt and pepper and mix well.

2 Take your sausage skins and rinse them in water. Push
a metal funnel into the end of one skin and tie a knot in
the other end. Push the meat mixture through the funnel
using the handle of a wooden spoon (make sure this can
pass right through the nozzle of the funnel). Keep pushing
the meat through the tube, easing it down with your hands,
until you have the size of sausage you want. Twist the skin,
tie a knot and cut it off. Repeat the process until you have
filled all the skins. This may seem laborious, but you will
get into it.

3 To cook your sausages, either fry them in a hot pan
with a little olive oil for about 15–20 minutes or put them
in an oven preheated to 180°C/Gas 4 for about 30 minutes.
An important thing to remember about homemade
sausages is that, without preservatives, they will only
stay fresh for 2 days, so eat them quickly!

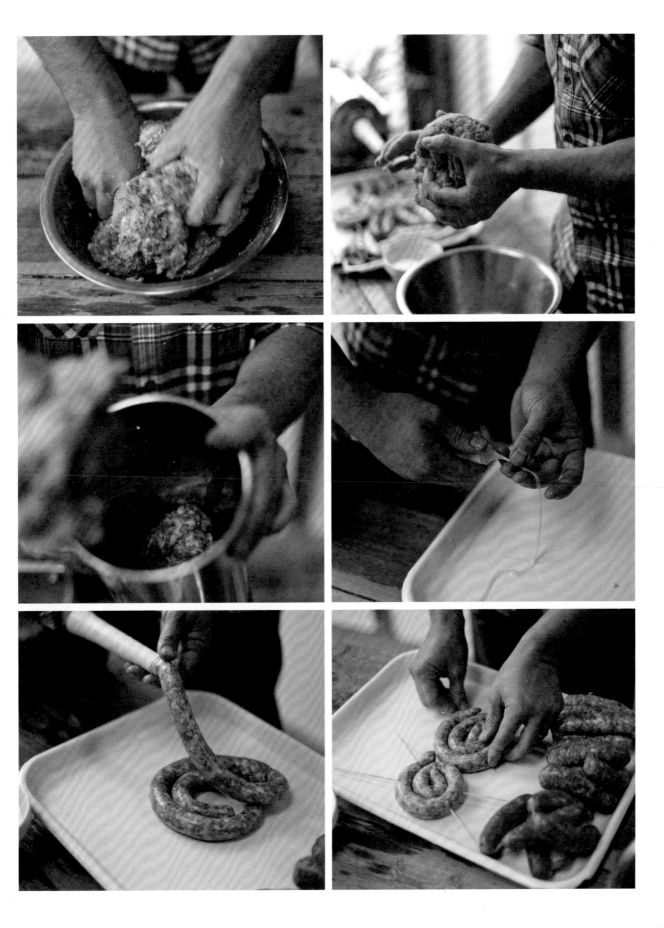

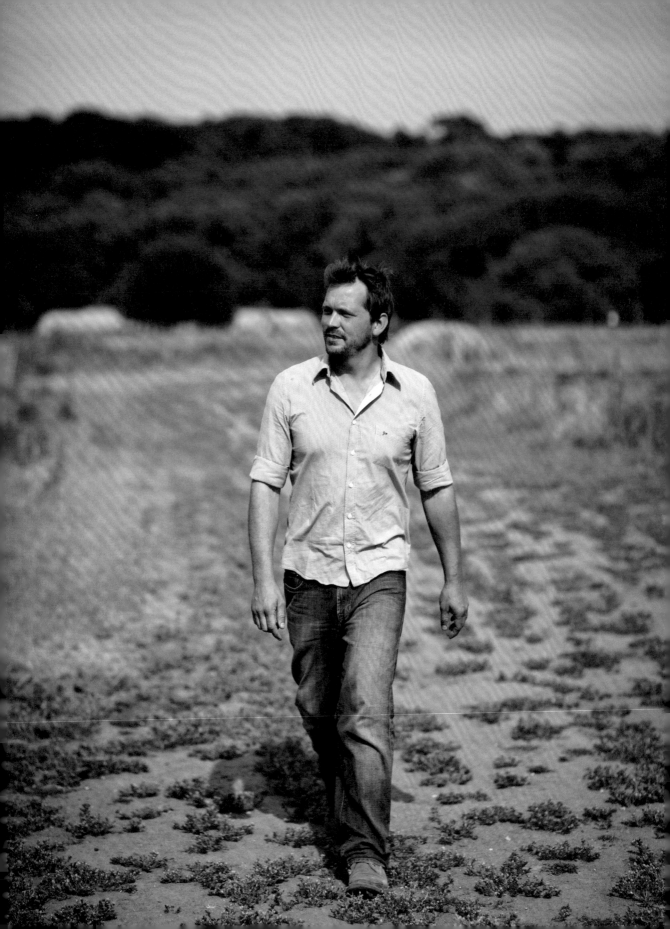

Useful contacts

General

The Department of Environment, Food and Rural Affairs (DEFRA) is the most important official body covering all aspects of cultivation and husbandry. As well as legislating on food issues, it has a wealth of helpful information on its website (ww2.defra.gov.uk) – and it's well worth looking into the wide range of grants available for everything from farming to conservation.

Local councils have jurisdiction over a wide range of farming activities. Some livestock – such as pigs – need to be registered with the Trading Standards Department and you will need a movement licence when picking them up and taking them to the abattoir. Talk to Environmental Health officers before processing food. New polytunnels and animal shelters may need planning permission.

The National Farmers Union (NFU) can be very helpful on a huge range of farming issues (www.nfuonline.com).

The Farming and Wildlife Advisory Group (FWAG) is great on environmental and conservation issues (www.fwag.org.uk).

If you are interested in selling your produce, the National Farmers' Retail and Markets Association is a good starting point (www.farma.org.uk).

There are several organisations which give you the accreditation to allow you to sell your produce as organic. The Soil Association (www.soilassociation.org) is the oldest, but Organic Farmers and Growers (www.organicfarmers.org.uk) is bigger.

If you want to have a look at how I've put together my own answers to the problems of making a living from food production in modern Britain, my farm near Ipswich welcomes visitors (www.jimmysfarm.com).

Animals

There are a host of clubs dedicated to specific animals, but the Rare Breeds Survival Trust is a good starting point and has a wealth of information on threatened livestock (see www.rbst.org.uk).

The British Hen Welfare Trust is always looking for homes for spent hens and also provides excellent advice advice on how to keep them (www.bhwt.org.uk).

The British Beekeepers Association (www.britishbee.org.uk–National Beekeeping Centre, Stoneleigh Park, Warwickshire CV5 2LG).

Growing

The Henry Doubleday Research Association has a Heritage Seed Library which supplies members with otherwise unobtainable plant varieties (www.gardenorganic.org.uk) while the French Association Kokopelli does the same (www.terredesemences.com).

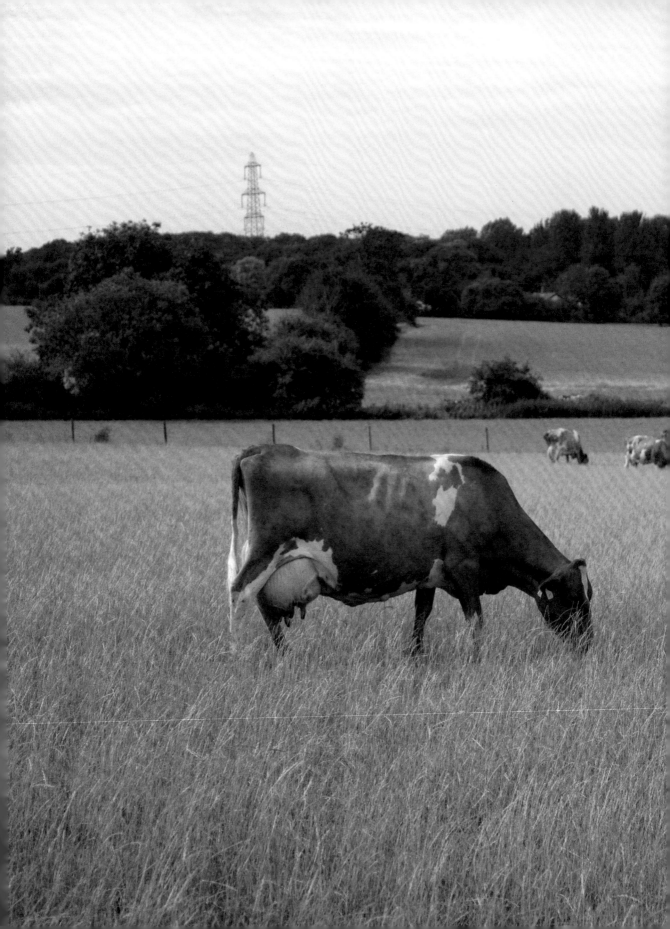

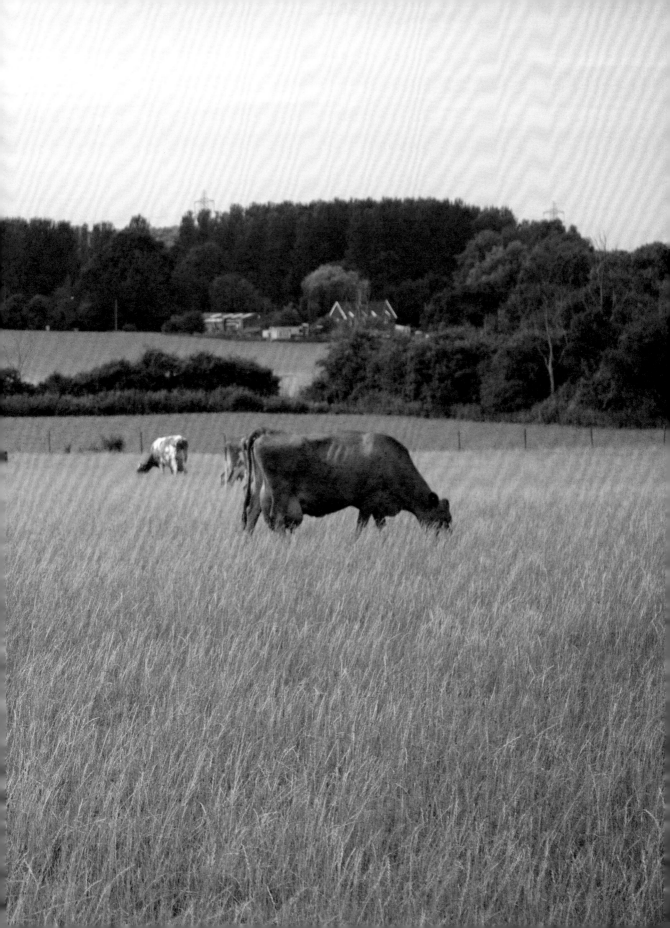

Index

Acknowledgements

Big Thanks to:

Jenny Heller, Simon Gerratt, Georgina Atsiaris and Helena Caldon and the rest of the team at HarperCollins for helping this book come to life. To Jane Lush, Fenia Vardanis, Ian Holt, Kate Gibbard and the rest of the team at Splash Media.

Daniel Butler for all your help with the book.

A massive thank you to Chris Terry for his fabulous photography.

My team at Fresh Partners, Debbie Catchpole, Verity O'Brien and Kelly Enfield for all their support. To Louise Plank and Beverly Comboy at Plank PR.

A very special thanks to everyone at Jimmy's Farm for your constant hard work.

Also a big cheers to Paul Kelly at Kelly Bronze Turkeys.

And last but not least, to those behind the scenes: Stephen Maynard and Nikki Morgan. My wonderful wife Michaela and beautiful daughter Molly.

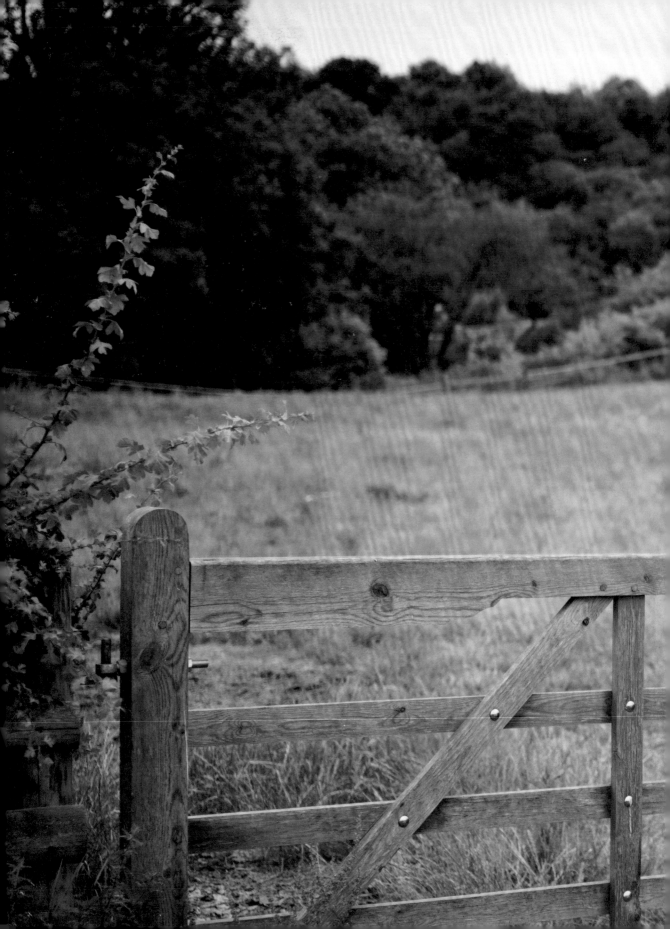

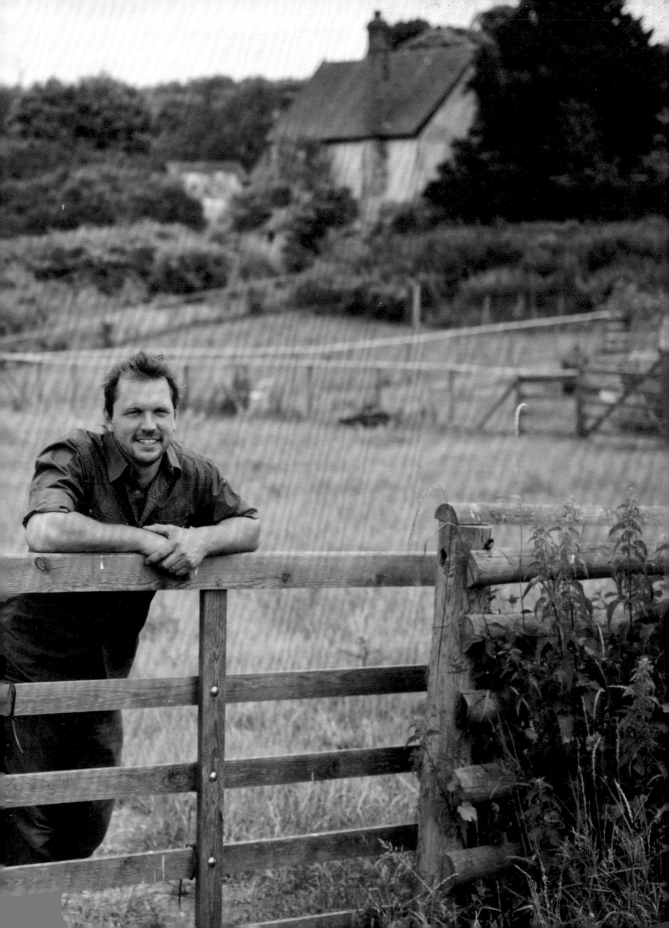

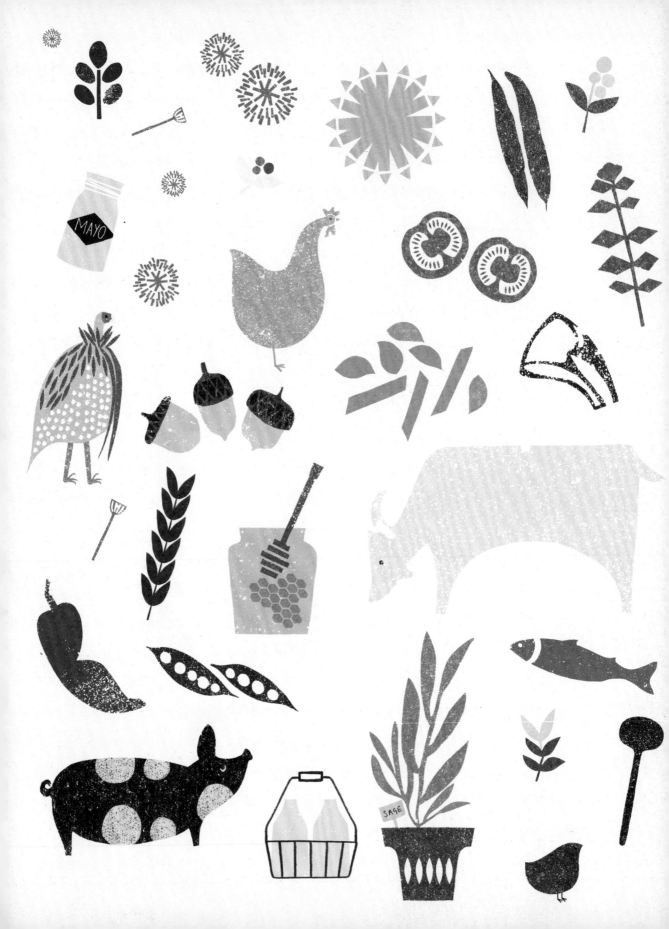